Praise for Rising UP!

For more information, please visit www.annayork.com.

Read Rising UP!. You will be both inspired and edified… It tells how Anna York brought together Eastern (Tai Chi) and Christian spiritual practices to heal herself and create New Creation Body Prayer, the program that is used in churches and hospitals to help others. This book will get under your skin and into your heart. I highly recommend it.
—Don Browning, Alexander Campbell Professor, University of Chicago Divinity School, Emeritus, and author of *Reviving Christian Humanism: The New Conversation on Theology, Spirituality, and Psychology*

When we pick up this book, we are in store for more than a good read—we are on the brink of an adventure. Our guide is Anna York, who is herself a multi-dimensional person, and the terrain is the several worlds in which she has taken up citizenship. She leads us into the deep and challenging places of these worlds—her amazing personal engagement with multiple sclerosis, her profound personal and spiritual journey, her "easternizing" her journey through tai chi and Chinese medicine, and her struggle to synthesize these element with her western and Christian identity, all the while moving steadily toward her professional goals and ministry. But there is more to her story than any summary can convey—surprising turns, puzzling conundrums, and thrilling discovery. This is the kind of book that goes beyond information and inspiration—it transforms us.
—Philip Hefner, Lutheran Pastor and Professor Emeritus of Systematic Theology at the Lutheran School of Theology at Chicago.

Rising UP! is a valuable addition to narratives about life with disability, and in particular how one woman, after unsuccessfully navigating the traditional medical and religious structures, ultimately finds unexpected and creative solutions back to health and well-being.
 —Kristi L. Kirschner M.D., Physical Medicine and Rehabilitation

As Anna's pastor for fourteen years I shared her struggle for healing in an intellectual, spiritual, multi-cultural melting pot. She discovers that Christ does not always answer prayers in the way we expect. He is as iconoclastic now as he was in his own day, breaking down religious and cultural barriers and compelling us to see God at work in the world around us. Anna inspires all of us to persevere in seeking healing for ourselves and peace for our world.
 —Rev. Dr. Shanta Premawardhana, Executive for Interreligious Dialogue and Cooperation at the World Council of Churches

*I hope the story of my journey
and my recovery will help you with yours.*

Rising UP!

My Recovery from Multiple Sclerosis, Disability and Despair

by

Anna York

Rising UP!
My Recovery from Multiple Sclerosis, Disability and Despair

© 2010 Anna York
All Rights Reserved. Published 2010
17 16 15 14 13 12 11 10   1 2 3 4 5

ISBN: 978-0-9763675-8-1

Published by First Flight Books
A division of Bruce Bendinger Creative Communications, Inc.
2144 N. Hudson • Chicago, IL 60614
773-871-1179 • FX 773-281-4643

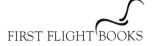

Book Design: Patrick Aylward
Cover Design: Gregory S. Paus

No part of this publication may be reproduced or transmitted in any form or by any means electronic or mechanical, including photocopy, recording or any information storage and retrieval system now known or to be invented, without permission in writing from the copyright owner, except by a reviewer who wishes to quote brief passages in connection with a review written for inclusion in a magazine, newspaper, broadcast or website.

Neither the author nor the publisher is engaged in rendering professional advice or services to the individual reader. The ideas and suggestions contained in this book are not intended as a substitute for consulting with your physician. All matters regarding health require medical supervision. Neither the author nor the publisher shall be liable or responsible for any loss, injury, or damage allegedly arising from any information or suggestion in this book.

For further information, visit the author's website:
www.annayork.com

Dedication

*This book is dedicated to my students
and to friends everywhere who are Rising UP!
in the face of impossible odds to find healing and wholeness.*

*Gerald, Leigh, Al, Barbara, Eve, Fred, Mary, Jane,
Maureen, Jeanne, Larry, Flora, Mike, Lenore—
and so many more!—this is for you.*

Author's Note

This book has been in the making for twenty years, encountering many wonderful supporters and several roadblocks on its journey to publication. I have learned that a baby is born when the time is right. Some people who have helped with birthing this book deserve special mention. I could not have written *Rising UP!* without the incredible support and love of my husband Don. Bruce Moran, in addition to serving as a teacher, trainer and friend, read and commented extensively on the text. Shanta Premawardhana, my pastor for fourteen years and friend of twenty years, gave me insight, wisdom, and courage at all times. Stephen Casari, my agent for seven years, believed in my book from the beginning. I am grateful to the many people who have read and commented and encouraged me along the way, including Dr. Kristi Kirschner, Professor Don Browning, Professor Phil Hefner, Rev. Susan Johnson, Scott McDonald, Rev. David Kyllo, and my own sons, Sean, Maurice, Chandler and Jeremy.

Thanks to the people at Bruce Bendinger Creative Communications who helped publish my book, especially Lorelei Davis Bendinger for her inspired guidance, Patrick Aylward for the book design, and Greg Paus for the beautiful cover.

I have changed some names in my story to protect privacy.

Contents

Introduction: I AM One	1
The Rising Heritage	
My Name is Anna	9
Growing Up Fundamentalist	15
Falling Down	
Dorothy in Kansas	35
Signs in the Heavens, Signs in the Earth	42
Moving Out in Spirit	47
I Feared a Fear	55
The Price of Liberty	57
Doing, Doing, Doing Too Much	61
Our Little Girl Dies	66
The Fear Came Upon Me	67
Do-Be-Do-Be-Do	72
Will Power Is Not Enough	76
Future Shock	84
Demolition of the Past	88
Denial of the Present	91
Alone and Lonely	94
Does Anybody Know This Person?	99
Victimized	102
Unknowing	105
Seeking Who I AM	
Seeking the Way	113
Finding "The Way"	118
Being Who I Am	122
Who I Am as Myself	125
Being Empty and Full	132
Meeting the "I AM"	140

A Rising Manifesto

A Mountaintop Experience	145
Snowstorm	147
I AM Faith	152
Window Watcher	158
I AM Joy	161
Never Christmas	166
I AM Hope	169
Broken Neck	177
I AM Love	180

Rising and Falling

Up and Down the Mountain	189
Coming Together	194
Everybody's Mom	201
Parking Violations	205
The Man in My Life	208
Flashes in My Soul	217

Rising UP!

Jubilee	225
I Am Who I AM: Preparing for Ordination	230
Riding the Wind, Serving Tea: Ordination	233
Waving Palms: Healed by a Tai Chi Master	239
Born Again	245
Tai Chi: Exercise I Could Do	248
Easternizing My Healing	261
A Grace Place Healing	265
Food for Life	271
Walking Free!	280
A Traditional Chinese Medicine Diagnosis	286
Drug Free!	293
Body Prayer	300

Detoxing the Emotions	309
Roaring and Forgiving	314
Chi and Other Dilemmas	320
Clearing Out, Moving On	328
Cutting the Strings	334
The Falling Icon	342
Adventures and Vistas	347
Rising Costs	353
Photo Album	361
Epilogue	
New Year, 2010	373

Introduction
I Am One

My husband Don says I'm non-statistical. Since he is a chaired Professor of Astrophysics at the University of Chicago and has hundreds of scientific papers to his credit, I figure he should know. One of his favorite pastimes is calculating in his head, on the spur of the moment, such complex questions as the budget of a corporation, the resources needed for putting computers in every room of the Chicago Public Schools, the population of the world 50 years from now and the number of atoms in the universe. He calculates my personal non-statistical status by citing the following criteria: I have MS (one in a thousand); I am a vegan (he only knows three others in the world); I am a female Baptist minister (a species on the endangered list); I am a female Baptist minister who does Tai Chi (a set of one, as far as he knows); and I am a female Baptist minister with multiple sclerosis who has recovered with the help of a Tai Chi master (the only one in the universe). All of these peculiarities together make it impossible for me to share a category with anyone else; therefore, I am "non-statistical."

Even though Don loves me unconditionally—and has proven it by sticking it out with me for all these years!—my non-statistical status is still puzzling to him. He depends on statistics and data to make measurements, interpretations and predictions about what is happening and can happen in the physical universe. In Don's view, if there is just one event of a particular kind, there is no way to determine whether it is a random anomaly, an experimental error, or an indicator that there is a whole dimension of reality that is as yet unknown and unexplored and that waits on the horizon to be discovered. Scientifically, these kinds of questions fascinate him, and he's built a career trying to make sense of them. Maybe that's why he finds me fascinating and has stayed with me—I am one more mystery of the universe yet to be solved! Here are some of the facts he's assembled in his attempt to understand my experience:

- I have had multiple sclerosis since 1965 (about 45 years as of this writing!) and was severely crippled for over a decade. Up to six MS attacks a year resulted in my using an electric scooter and being unable to stand or sit up straight for more than a few minutes.
- I was largely paralyzed in my lower left body and the muscles all over my body were atrophied.
- At times my hands were so weak I was unable to lift a cup or plate.
- While there are now drugs that help reverse the symptoms of MS, there is still no known cure, and many fight a losing battle to control their symptoms. I have not only controlled but also reversed mine, finding healing in body, mind and spirit.
- I am no longer using a scooter or even a cane, and my physical exams reveal excellent overall health. After being uninsurable for more than two decades, I have now been approved for life insurance! I stand straight and tall and fit into my wedding dress (45 years and 5 babies ago).
- I live a normal life, work 40 hours a week and love to travel and work out.

Don has seen me go through a lot of changes. No wonder he's puzzled.

There are also others who are challenged by my non-statistical status. When I last saw my neurologist, in 2002, I had to register as a new patient because I had not seen him for so long. I wanted him to see my progress. He listened with raised eyebrows and then pronounced my current healthy status as being "lucky"—another way of saying "non-statistical." My experience does not fit the normal categories of healing in the Western medical framework because I have broken out of it and departed into the unscientific and "anecdotal" world of natural, alternative, and complementary healing. Because my doctor does not have any data to support a regimen such as mine, he cannot bring himself to say that my "good luck" will continue or that it might be a possibility for anyone else.

Some people say I am a miracle, which is yet another way of saying I am non-statistical. This often happens with people who are not religious. They just go by their seat-of-the-pants observations that something has occurred that seems completely out of the range of normal experience. For these people, wide eyes and a sense of awe often accompany their perception of my miraculous status.

Those who are Christians, especially those who are from conservative backgrounds like mine, hesitate to call me a miracle, because my experience does not fit what they recognize as a canonical, Biblical healing. It did not fall on me instantaneously from on high but has taken place over a period of years and is still taking place today. Furthermore, even though the prayers of hundreds of people were instrumental in bringing about my healing, and even though one important healing occurred in a church sanctuary, much of my healing was accomplished in my home and in Tai Chi classes and workout gyms. Nor was it performed by a traditional "minister" or church "healer" but primarily through the expertise of a Tai Chi master who is highly skilled in Eastern healing arts. For some Christians, including some who are very close to me, these circumstances are disturbing and confusing. Part of my story is about my struggle to share my unusual experience with my Christian friends and loved ones.

From my own perspective, I do think of myself as a miracle. The Bible says that some miracles need to be "worked"— which means that a great deal of energy or *dunamis* (the Greek word from which we get our word "dynamite") goes into creating something extraordinary. My experience has been a "dynamite" miracle of faith, hope, will, discipline, insight, adaptation and transformation. While it has been God working in me to accomplish the miracle, I have also been a co-creative partner, along with other people from outside my own religious faith and milieu who I never expected could participate in such a work of God. The miracle is not finished. I will be working it every day, day in and day out, for the rest of my life. Living means working miracles, never stopping, never giving up, rebuking the impossible, grasping God's new possibilities, snatching life from death, rising up to live again.

While the story of how I received physical healing is important, I believe it has broader implications. It is a sign of hope, cooperation and understanding in our fractured, war-torn world. My experience is Western, but it breaks out of Western definitions and structures and speaks that we are not whole until we learn that the heritage of other cultures can be God's gift of love to us. I am a Christian, and my experience is deeply Christian, but God surprised me by breaking through frontiers of time and space, through walls between nations and people groups, through barriers of the heart and spirit. My experience bursts out of traditional Christian patterns and dogmas and recaptures some of the iconoclastic nature of Christ's original healing ministry. People of any faith, or no faith at all, can find hope in my story because it speaks once again, as it did in that ancient time, of a God who is great beyond all comprehension and whose love crosses all boundaries.

My journey has brought me from rural, fundamentalist roots in America's heartland to the pluralistic, urban setting where I have experienced healing through the Eastern arts. For me, this journey is as unlikely as traveling to the moon. It has transported me from the familiar, comfortable doctrines of my childhood faith into the heart center and offense of Christ's gospel—the gospel that there is a new humanity and that the walls of hostility are broken down among all people so that we may seek and discover the meaning of God's love among all the diverse expressions of those who are created in God's own image. It has taken me away from a passive, yielded faith to an active, co-creative participation in community with people of diverse nations and faiths. Within that community I commit myself to struggle and wrestle with the meaning of our similarities and differences and to assist each other in finding healing and mutual transformation so that we can have peace in our world.

My non-statistical status proclaims that I AM ONE. My story is unique. Even so, the fact that I have a unique story suggests to me that there is a whole world full of unique stories out there, if only we could tune in to hear them all. By sharing our stories we affirm to each other that even though there is anguish, loss and pain, there is also the possibility of hope, power and transformation. We say to each other, "No matter how bad things may seem, there is always hope. If I can get through it, you can too." I AM ONE with all such stories that can and will be. Let us rise up together and share the journey.

The "Rising" Heritage

My Name is Anna

My name is Anna. Years ago, in a moment of inner quiet at an altar call, I heard my name spoken softly, *"Your name is Anna. It means 'the grace of God.'"* I did not realize at the time that it would be grace that would define who I am, my path, my purpose, my destiny.

My spiritual roots run deep. On the paternal side we trace our roots on the American continent to William and Margaret Hind, who arrived at the Jamestown colony on a ship named *Paule* from London, on July 6, 1635, less than thirty years after the Jamestown colony was founded. These hearty pioneers were followed by numerous other Hind families, Scots-Irish Presbyterians who were willing to face harsh living in a new land in order to have religious freedom. Some of them moved from Jamestown to the Great Valley of Virginia, where there is a record of another William Hind being baptized with his children, William Jr. and Margaret, at the Tinkling Spring church in the Augusta Colony in 1749. Succeeding generations moved on to Kentucky around the time of Daniel Boone, and, once again, it is baptisms and church membership that document the life of my ancestors. Our branch of the Hind family settled in the Blue River area of Washington County in Indiana. The earliest record I have found of the name changing to "Hinds" is around 1837 with my great grandfather, James Pleasant Hinds, who passed the new spelling down to all succeeding generations in our branch of the family.

For as far back as the records go, our people have been humble, godly folk, living close to the land and close to their Creator. My father's cousin, Ethel Sullivan, a tiny, bird-like spinster with sparkling eyes and wispy red hair, wrote a family history that includes this as a motto that fits the Hinds family well:

> "To live as gently as I can;
> To be a friend to every man;
> To take what comes of good or ill,
> And cling to faith and honor still;

And then, should failure come to me,
Still work and hope for victory." —Anonymous

On the maternal Neal side, which is less clearly documented, the forbears were also godly folk, bearing among their ranks faithful, hardworking souls who loved God and their fellowman. The heritage of faith passed down through the generations to the post World War II Baby Boom generation into which I was born in 1945.

I share the name Anna with my paternal grandmother, Anna Goforth Hinds, a woman of pioneering spirit who lovingly served as wife to Horace Pleasant Hinds, an itinerant gospel preacher, and who nurtured six children through two world wars and the Great Depression. Anna Goforth was the mother of Ariel, later to become my father. One of my favorite stories about her is her valiant effort to save my father's leg from amputation when he was only sixteen years old. Ariel was filling the gas tank of their Model T Ford along the side of a country road when a drunk driver crashed into him, pinning his leg between the two cars. The doctor recommended amputation for his mangled limb. Anna Goforth insisted that her son needed two good legs to get through life, and she refused permission for the doctor to cut off the leg. She fought for her son to be whole against impossible odds, and her persistence paid off. My father walked on two legs throughout his long life to the ripe old age of 94. I have always believed that I capture much of my Rising spirit from Anna Goforth.

My Grandpa, Horace Pleasant, also had a major impact on me. The imposing square jaw and hooked nose I see in his pictures belie a kind, gentle man who was devoted to his family and to serving the Lord. His true calling was ministry, and he traveled around central Indiana on weekends to serve as preacher for numerous small congregations. During the week he scratched out

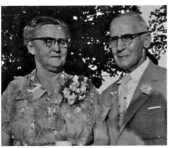
My grandparents, Anna Goforth and Horace Pleasant Hinds

a living by farming. In my archive of family pictures there is a yellowed photograph of one of their earlier homes, a humble, gray clapboard farm cottage near Gosport, Indiana. He was a great lover of books and eventually assembled a large library that covered a wide range of the theological and philosophical issues of his day. He carefully hand bound many of his volumes and annotated them in an elegant, flowing script.

When my sisters and I divided the family heirlooms, I inherited Grandpa's briefcase full of sermons and notes. I discovered that he outlined his sermons the same way I do—I didn't know a thing like that could run in the genes. He also visualized his sermons with charts and graphic designs that he would paint on white bed sheets and hang on the wall behind the pulpit, an early precursor to the PowerPoint and digital graphics I use today. Grandpa was not a wealthy man, but he considered it worthwhile to purchase one of the early Underwood typewriters to type his sermons. He taught himself how to type and took time to highlight important points by moving the ribbon from black to red for emphasis and back again to black for regular text. I remember him sitting at his typewriter in deep thought with a green plastic visor to shield his eyes from incoming sunlight. He typed on the back side of shopping lists, handbill advertising and any other scrap of paper he could find in order to conserve precious resources. When I handle these browning notes today, I feel his love and dedication flowing to me in the very paper and ink with which the words are written.

As I grew up, Grandpa Hinds was the closest I could get to imagining what God is like. If I ever thought of doing something questionable, I would think of Grandpa, and then I would change my mind and do what I thought he would approve. Even after he died, his moral influence was strong until I was a grown woman with my first child. I recall thinking at that time, "Well, Grandpa, I'm old enough now. Maybe it's time for me to trust God to help me make my own decisions. But I know you'll always be there." I felt he was smiling at me and letting me know he would always love me.

Ariel Hinds, my father, captured the Rising spirit from his parents and manifested it throughout his life. He was a self-educated man whose creativity, optimism and humor sustained all of us through both good times and bad times. I grew up on a farm, and sometimes things happened there that no one could control, such as the heavy rains that came booming down the valley, flooding the bottomland and destroying our crops. I remember my father watching in tears from the porch window as the water swept across the bottom cornfield and washed all his labor away. But somehow he always rebounded. He used his ingenuity to tile the lowlands and get control of the water. He kept right on planting, year after year, and each harvest was greater than the one before.

Daddy was able to change with the times. When the expense of equipment and maintenance took too big a chunk out of the income and debt began to pile up, he bought himself a bulldozer and contracted out for construction work, an enterprise that kept us afloat economically for several years.

One of the most formative examples of Rising power that my father set for me was the amazing transformation after the heart attack he had at age 59. The attack, brought on by shoveling snow away from the door of the garage, was so devastating that for a long time afterward he walked with difficulty and was unable to climb stairs. He knew he would no longer be able to do his life-long work of farming, so he reinvented himself, switching careers in circumstances that would have made many people roll over and go belly up. He sold the farm, moved into town, took all the qualifying tests, and became a realtor.

As he began his new business, he struggled with pain and weakness and always carried nitro tablets in his pocket to protect himself in case of frequent, severe angina. Since he could not climb stairs, he and Mother renovated their house and put an elevator in it, a most unusual feature for a residence in that rural area. It looked to everyone like his condition was permanent and that he would have a short, painful life.

Amazingly, a wonderful spiritual renewal burst forth in his life. He turned his eyes toward the Lord, and his faith became stronger and stronger. Finally one day he said, "God is closer than my chest pocket. I'm not going to carry these pills any more!" And he didn't! From that time, his health improved, along with his love and devotion for the Lord. He walked the hills of southern Indiana selling real estate, trekked away on hunting expeditions, and lived a full, joyous life. The elevator became a way of testifying to all my parents' guests about the wonderful grace of God in healing him and giving him a long, vigorous life. As he ripened into old age, surviving all of his immediate family and most of his contemporaries in the community, he would say with a twinkle in his eye, "I don't have any enemies. I outlived them all." His ability to renew himself through faith in God has been a guiding light for the many times I have had to reinvent my own life. I expect, like him, to outlive everyone I know.

My mother, Audrey Ruth Hinds, was a hard act to follow, a good match for the loving husband to whom she was married for sixty years. She was a woman of boundless energy, enthusiasm and creativity. She was always up in the morning before everyone else, and she kept forging onward when the rest of us were too tired, too sick or too dispirited to go a step further. If we began to falter, she, with her indomitable spirit, would demand, "Get up from there and put a smile on your face!"—and she would lead the way with singing, usually a hymn such as "Onward, Christian Soldiers" or "Stand Up, Stand Up for Jesus." She knew how to use faith and theology for practical purposes!

Wherever Mother went, there was new life and creativity. She originated a new method of teaching children in groups called the SMV method—for the Social, Mental and indiVidual charac-

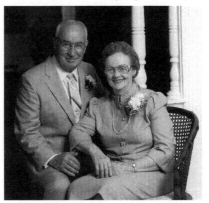

My wonderful parents, Audrey and Ariel Hinds.

teristics of each child. Her first grade room became a demonstration classroom for schools all over the state. Alongside of her innovative educational methods, she quietly but powerfully engaged in a ministry of prayer and healing every day in her classroom, as well as in the community. One day a child came up to her with sniffles, and she touched him and said, "You're all right now"—and the child went away smiling. Another time she touched a child with crossed eyes and his eyes straightened out immediately, eliminating the need for surgery. Miracles were an everyday occurrence for my mother. She began a nursery school, a nursing home visitation program, and a prison ministry, all in addition to her legendary hospitality. She was able to throw together a meal for twelve on the spur of the moment, drawing on a freezer full of homemade casseroles, bird pies, and scrumptious desserts. Her joy overflowed into everything she did.

Sometimes when I am very quiet, I still think I can hear my mother singing, which she did at home, in the car, in her classroom—everywhere she went. Her legacy of love for God is attested in a shelf full of heavily underlined and annotated Bibles. She was the most purehearted person I ever hope to meet. When she was 75, she could run circles around me. All those who loved her marked her death with singing and celebration for the joy of knowing her and knowing that her soul flew straight to God's bosom.

My name is Anna. I came from good stock, from folks who knew how to rise and keep on rising.

Growing up Fundamentalist

All the people I knew in my family were people who loved the Lord. My uncle Immanuel was the preacher for our little congregation when I was growing up, and most of my male relatives were preachers, elders, deacons, and song leaders. My father was an elder, and some of my earliest memories are of him teaching Sunday school to all the children in our church. From oldest to youngest, we would sit on the front pew together, and he would start with Genesis 1 and work his way through the Bible verse by verse: "And now who can say the names of the twelve tribes of Israel . . . . ?" I dangled my short legs off the edge of the hard, oak-plank bench and tried to answer as many questions as my older sister and cousins—"Reuben, Simeon, Levi, Judah, Gad, Asher . . ." We learned to sing all the books of the Old and New Testaments and all the twelve apostles' names—and so much more!

Our family life on the farm was also focused on the Lord. We said prayers reverently three times a day at meals—blessing the food was as important as eating it. On cold winter evenings we would curl up in warm jammies and blankets for devotionals and Bible readings around the hot-air vent in the dining room, the room closest to the furnace and the coziest place in the house. We would say family prayers and would also pray our own individual prayers before going to bed. God was intertwined in the most fundamental acts of life, part of our food and breath.

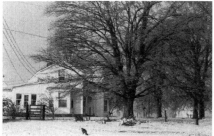

The farmhouse where I grew up near Worthington, Indiana.

The True Church

I attended the Church of Christ, the church that several generations of my family before me attended. Sometime in the early 1800's in Kentucky, a man named Thomas Campbell led a group of believers who desired to be known as "Christians only" away from the Presbyterians, the denomination that was home to our family for many generations. One group of the "Campbellites" became the Disciples of Christ and another became the Church of Christ. My family on both sides were Church of Christ people, probably dating back to the mid nineteenth century.

Our home congregation was located on a corner lot on Jefferson Street in Worthington, Indiana, on land that my Grandpa Hinds donated. Our church believed that it was imperative to worship just as the early church did and that we had succeeded in restoring the ancient ways after hundreds and thousands of years of other people going astray. My uncle Earl wrote a scholarly treatise on this subject entitled *The Search for the Ancient Order*.

We Church of Christers did not regard ourselves as a "denomination," a term which we thought implied being an offshoot of the Catholic Church, but as the "true" church that Jesus established in the first century. This was reflected in our name, "Church of Christ," in which "Church" represents not a denomination or individual church but the only *true* church. We were proud of our name because it identified us as followers of Christ rather than as adherents to Presbyterianism,

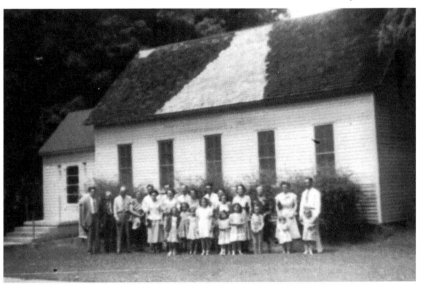

The Church of Christ in Worthington Indiana circa 1950. My parents are at the far right end with me and my sister Ruth. My sister Peggy and my cousins are in the center front.

Methodism and other denominations to which we attached the suffix "ism," which denoted that they had departed from the true way. "Ism" for us was something like "ites" in the Old Testament. The Hittites, Perizites, Hivites, Jebusites, Amalekites—and all the other "ites"—were tribes who did not know the true way of God and were destined to be conquered by the chosen people of Israel. The fact that the Presbyterians had the "ism" attached was an indication that by the time I arrived on the scene our family had long forgotten that it was that venerable denomination that brought us to this land, settled us in it and nourished us from earliest colonial times.

We believed there are certain specific practices that are clearly exemplified in scripture and that the scriptures should always be followed to the letter. We quoted "book, chapter and verse" to prove our points, and we regarded those who did not follow these practices, including members of other Protestant denominations, as "lost." The Catholics were the worst, and we thought most if not all of them were going to hell. When we studied Revelation, we interpreted the Catholic Church as being the whore on the Seven Hills of Rome. We wanted to avoid doing anything the way Catholics did, for example kneeling, crossing ourselves or using "vain repetitions" like reciting the rosary. After a teaching on this one Sunday, I remember raising my eyebrows and thinking amusingly to myself that we should be coming into the church through the windows because Catholics always enter through the doors. Of course I never said it out loud!

Next worst after the Catholics were the "holy rollers" (Pentecostals) who were undoubtedly possessed by the devil because they spoke in tongues. God only knew what other abominations they must practice! Those were the days prior to Pope John XXIII and Vatican II, and there was little inter-denominational and inter-faith dialogue, especially in the rural areas of the midwestern heartland. We had low tolerance for those who believed and worshiped differently than we did.

With so many people being "lost," there was a great need for evangelism. This was a heavy burden to bear on our shoulders, considering that everyone in the entire world was doomed if we did not bring them the true gospel. Every little church that had a revival was doing so to "save the world." Perhaps this impossible yet imperative task, coupled with unquestioning optimism and faith, helped to imbue me with the belief that there is nothing impossible with God, a belief that would stand me in good stead later in life.

The Bible as the Word of God

Our God was one who is revealed in the Bible, the inspired Word of God. We believed the canon of scripture is complete and that God has said all he will ever say in the Bible as we have it today. For this reason, we thought it was of greatest importance to study the Bible and interpret it correctly. Certain words from Revelation were often cited as a warning that nothing should be used as a guide except the Bible: "I warn everyone who hears the words of the prophecy of this book; if anyone adds to them, God will add to that person the plagues described in this book; if anyone takes away from the words of the book of this prophecy, God will take away that person's share in the tree of life and in the holy city, which are described in this book." Just have a look and you will see that the plagues are pretty horrible, including "foul and painful sores," scorching by fierce heat, and people who "gnaw their tongues in agony"—none of which I wanted to happen to me! When the Revelator referred to the prophecy of "this book," we took it to mean not just the book of Revelation but the whole Bible, Old and New Testaments, as we knew it. Of course we excluded the Apocrypha, which was one of those forbidden additions to the true Word. The fact that Catholics, Presbyterians, Methodists and others had prayer books in addition to the Bible was cited as an indication that they were on the path to the fiery pit. Hell was fire and brimstone and gnashing of teeth. I was sorry for the Presbyterians and Methodists, but not especially for the Catholics because I didn't know any of them. Ours was a strongly Protestant community.

Baptism by Immersion

We believed that the only way to be properly baptized is by complete immersion in water, and that only people old enough to make a true profession of faith could be baptized. For this reason, we thought that those who practiced infant baptism or baptism by sprinkling or pouring were placing their souls in eternal jeopardy.

Since we regarded baptism as the way one becomes a Christian and thus enters into the blessings of the kingdom of God, baptismal services were holy events. A few churches had baptisteries, but we baptized outdoors as often as possible. Sometimes we would all gather on the banks of the pond that my father built with his bulldozer on our farm. It was a peaceful place a short distance behind the old red barn, surrounded by fields of corn and woodlands. We would reverently sing hymns such as "The Old Rugged Cross" and "What Can Wash Away My Sin? Nothing but the Blood of Jesus." Reverent voices lifted in humble faith floated upward into a blue sky.

We believed that all believers were equal in the sight of God and that anyone could perform a baptism, but it was usually the preacher who officiated. While we sang, the preacher and the baptismal candidate would wade through the mud and cattails to a depth that allowed convenient immersion. The preacher would put his hand on the shoulder of the candidate and say, "Mary, do you believe Jesus Christ is the Son of God?" Then, on hearing the confession, "I do," he would raise his right hand and say, "I now baptize you in the name of the Father, the Son and the Holy Ghost." Holding a handkerchief over the nose and mouth, he would lay the person backward and down into the water. The person would come up sputtering and soaking wet but with a glowing smile, knowing her soul was now safe. As the candidate came up out of the water, we would sing "Just as I am, without one plea, but that thy blood was shed for me." I can still hear the sweet, tearful voices, raised in four-part harmony, and feel the warmth of heart we all shared together. Those were sacred, reverent times as we ushered souls into newness of life.

I myself was baptized at about the age of 10, but since it was cool weather, it was not a good time to use the pond. I was immersed by my Grandpa Hinds in a baptistery in the Church of Christ in Coal City, Indiana, a tiny town a few miles away from our farm. Coal City is named for the strip coal mining that plowed up the whole countryside around there, right up to the village boundaries. We watched from our school bus daily as the gargantuan stripper shovel chewed away the earth like an apocalyptic monster, laying the land to waste. The town survives today, possibly due to the never-say-die spirit of its residents, which is captured on the city limit sign as you enter town: "Coal City. 213 Happy Souls and One Old Grouch."

The red brick Church of Christ with a simple white spire is still there on the outskirts next to a cornfield. The baptistery in which I was baptized is in an alcove behind the pulpit. In my youth it had a lovely painting of a blue river with green banks and weeping willows. The tank was always filled with water in case a soul should express a desire to be saved during the gospel invitation at the end of each service. A red velvet curtain was drawn across the front before each baptism so people wouldn't see the candidates going down into the water, and the pulpit was taken to the side so the congregation could view the event. On the day I was baptized I went down into the water with my Grandpa as we heard the congregation singing,

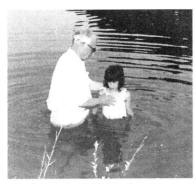

My father, Ariel Hinds, baptizing my niece Kirsten in the pond on the Davis family farm, circa 1987.

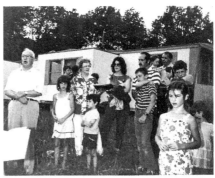

The family sings on the banks of the pond before the baptism.

O happy day that fixed my choice
On Thee, my Savior and my God!
Well may this glowing heart rejoice,
And tell its raptures all abroad!
Happy day, happy day,
When Jesus washed my sins away.

Then the curtains opened, and Grandpa said in a tender voice, his eyes soft and gentle: "Anna Sue, do you believe Jesus Christ is the Son of God?"

I answered, "Yes," and he laid me back under the water, marking the beginning of my lifelong commitment to Jesus. My cousin Miriam, who is the same age I am, was baptized on the same day.

The Lord's Supper

All Churches of Christ agreed about the mode of baptism, but there were disagreements about other things that caused some churches to "withdraw" or "disfellowship" those who didn't hone to their particular interpretations of scripture. An example was the practice of the Lord's Supper. We all took it every Sunday because scripture says the early believers came together on the "first day of the week"— not every day and not just once a month as some denominations were in the habit of doing. The mode of serving, however, was a matter of contention. When I was young, some churches felt strongly that it should be served with just one cup because it clearly says in the Bible that the Lord took "the" cup. This was our practice for some years when I was growing up, and I still have, as part of my inheritance, the pressed glass goblet that was passed around among the faithful to partake of the emblem of the Lord's blood. Later, some congregations, including our own, decided it was doctrinally acceptable to serve it in a tray with a lot of little individual cups. Our local church was "liberal" or "enlightened" in this regard, and we felt sorry for the "one cuppers" who were so narrow minded.

We were all teetotalers, so we used unfermented grape juice for the Lord's Supper, believing that Jesus had also eschewed alcoholic beverages. We did not want to desecrate the Lord's body and blood by imbibing unholy spirits at the Lord's table. The fact that the Catholics used real wine was another sign they were on the path to perdition. As for the bread, we always used unleavened bread because at the Passover that is what Jesus would have used. I went to visit a Mormon church during my teen years and was shocked that they served pieces of something that looked like packaged Wonder bread. I was convinced it was a sign of false doctrine. I had that impression at least partly because of the form of bread we used at our church. For years one of the ladies in our congregation would make flat piecrust dough and score it with a knife so it could be easily chipped off in little tiny pieces. I always thought that the personal touch was something that helped make it special—and maybe a little more holy. Later we changed to the stale commercial crackers ordered from the church supply warehouse. I don't think Jesus used that kind either, but it was stiff and hard and that seemed to be the criterion. Unlike the Catholics, we received the bread and juice as "emblems," not as the actual body and blood of Christ. The communion table on which the emblems were served now resides in my living room as a treasured family heirloom.

Sunday School and Kitchens

The manner of education and use of the building were matters of contention among some churches. We believed it was okay to have Sunday school, a practice with which some churches did not agree. I'm not sure why, but I suspect it had to do with the need to "preach" the gospel, which seemed to mean standing behind a pulpit. My grandfather took a stand for Sunday school. When he deeded the property for our church building, he wrote into the legal document that the gift of the land was contingent on the church allowing Sunday school to be taught. If they stopped having Sunday school, the deed would revert to the original owner.

We were like most Churches of Christ in not having a kitchen in our building, because the Bible says that God's house is to be a place of prayer and worship. The scripture about the "den of thieves" and Jesus driving out the moneychangers was often associated with this subject, although I'm not sure why. It also says in I Corinthians 11:22, "Have you no homes of your own to eat and drink in?" which indicates you shouldn't make a meal out of it. We did have a practice of having very large Sunday dinners in our homes, complete with mashed potatoes and pot roast, to which we would invite visitors and other guests who came to church. Nowadays many Churches of Christ have kitchens and hardly anyone has the big Sunday dinners at home. While I don't mourn the kitchen doctrine, the home fellowship is quite a loss.

Sing It, Don't Play It

We did not believe in using instrumental music in church and believed that those who did so were astray from the true path. There was a lot of preaching on this subject, with many arguments from scripture. The main one was that the Apostle Paul admonished early Christians to sing "psalms, hymns and spiritual songs" and "make melody in their hearts" to the Lord (Colossians, 3:16). Since he didn't mention musical instruments, we should not presume to use them. We recalled that frightening passage in the book of Revelation that adding or subtracting from the book would result in eternal damnation. That warning was often cited as applying to instrumental music. Quite frankly, I was never able to reconcile that stern doctrine with the fact that King David played on his harp and that Psalm 150 plainly says to praise the Lord with trumpets, lutes and clanging cymbals! It seemed God had changed his mind somewhere along the way. It was also noticeable that "in church" and "out of church" were two different things. Some people had pianos at home for secular music but did not play hymns on them. We had a piano, and we did play hymns, but not when a group came over. I recall having a twinge of guilt about it once in a while, but, after all, I wasn't doing it in church! When there were so many rules, one sometimes had to make decisions about where they should start and stop.

The prohibition against musical instruments resulted in our learning to sing *a cappella* in parts. One of our favorite pastimes was to have "sings" at various people's houses and at gospel meetings and youth rallies around the area. Our family was pretty good at singing. My sisters and cousins often formed a group to sing such songs as "Out of the Ivory Palaces, into the World of Woe." I remember singing for many funerals, back in the days when there were still both old and young people in church together. One funeral song was "There'll be no more crepe on the doorknob, no funeral trains in the sky." Another was "Farther along, we'll know all about it. Farther, along, we'll understand why." Singing is an inheritance passed down to the generations. One of our favorite extended-family activities is still *a cappella* hymn singing, which all, even the grandchildren, do with great joy and gusto whenever there is a family gathering.

A White Male God

God was male. It wasn't something we discussed; it was just tacitly accepted in the same way that one accepts that water is wet and the sky is blue. When something is so obvious, there is no argument. The fact that God is male was the basis for the doctrine and practice that only men could take part in any leadership of the church and its worship. Scripture plainly said that women are the weaker sex. After all, Eve was the one who succumbed to the wiles of the Devil and then tempted Adam to sin. Thus, the burden of all sin since the beginning of the world rested on her shoulders.

The admonition for women to be in submission and not to take authority over men was frequently cited, although I can tell you there were no women storming the pulpit to push the men aside. We were thoroughly indoctrinated about our proper place. Men prayed, led the singing, preached, made announcements, and made all the decisions about church life and policy. Women taught children in Sunday school and Bible School, and I myself began teaching when I was in junior high. Females could not teach adult men at any time, although we could participate in discussions during Bible classes. Women fixed a lot of food and did most of the visitation and daily ministry. Even so, I had the feeling that men were the ones who did all the "important" things for God. For this reason, I harbored a secret wish to preach. The only outlet I had for my aspirations was to evangelize the cows in the barn lot, an activity that foreshadowed and possibly even helped me prepare for ministry years later. I would sit on top of the board fence by the barn and proclaim the Word of God vigorously to my bovine congregation. I expounded on Moses and the Ten Commandments, Elijah on Mount Carmel and Jonah and the whale. I quoted the Apostle Paul and admonished all to repent, be baptized and go to all nations to save the lost. I experimented with various gestures and elocutionary styles designed to get their attention and stir their souls. They would sleepily chew their cuds, shift their weight from one haunch to the other, pass gas, and stroll out of the barnyard before I issued the altar call. I never got the impression it would be easy!

As far as I knew, God was also white. There were no Negroes, Asians, or Hispanics in the rural Midwest to challenge the idea at that time, and the pictures all showed Jesus as white with blondish hair and blue eyes. When I was growing up there was an unwritten law that if a Negro stopped in town, he had to move on before nightfall. The Lyons Club still performed black-face minstrels into the early 1960's, and we all laughed uproariously at the shenanigans of the naive "darkies." Somehow, even though we sang "Jesus loves the little children, all the children of the world, red and yellow, black and white," we never connected it up with certain underlying assumptions in our own community. I never saw any black people until my junior high years when I went to Indianapolis to shop for my school clothes and saw them right there next to me in the elevator in L.S. Ayres!

Rapture and Resurrection

I grew up believing in Resurrection. It was the spiritual heritage from generations of fundamentalist forebears. The hope of eternal life in heaven was a core doctrine of our faith, pervading all of our Christian teaching. My grandfathers and uncles on both sides, my father, and other teachers taught me the Bible verse by verse from Genesis to Revelation, always with the goal of Resurrection in mind. Resurrection, first and foremost, had to do with the hope of going to heaven when we die. If we live according to the teachings of the Bible, being sure we do what it says, we will be rewarded with a life in heaven with Christ. Ideas of heaven were associated largely with images from St. John's Revelation and other portions of the Bible, but we especially grasped the images that fulfilled needs we had in our particular life situations. In the rather poor farming area in which I grew up, "streets of gold" was a popular image of heaven. People often requested our gospel quartet or choir to sing at funerals about walking streets of gold and about "No Tears in Heaven." Such images gave people the comfort and strength to go forward and bear the suffering and trials of life that seemed to overwhelm them here on earth. Envisioning heaven gave us hope that there is an end to suffering and that we will ultimately have life everlasting with Christ our Savior and God our Father.

Images of heaven were powerful motivators to live a holy life in the here and now. I heard many wonderful sermons on the beauty of heaven and how we will "live with Jesus evermore." Many of our family prayers ended with "and take us to heaven when we die." I grew up wanting to go to heaven and feeling it was the most worthy goal there was, especially if we could get some other people saved and take them along with us. Sermons about the beauty of heaven and the appeal to live righteously were especially effective when coupled with alternative pictures of fire and brimstone and the gnashing teeth of hell. I definitely didn't want to go there.

The hope of Resurrection was coupled with the belief that those who are true Christians will be "raptured" (suddenly caught up by Christ to heaven while still in the midst of living on the earth) and come back to reign with Christ for a thousand years, a time which we referred to as the Millennium. These blessed, chosen ones will avoid the terrible "tribulation" accompanying the apocalypse at the end of the world. Those who die in Christ will also be resurrected to reign with him. This view of the "end times" is called "pre-millennialism," and it was a topic so important that churches sometimes quarreled over the details, even disfellowshipping others that held a different view. My Grandpa Hinds preached Rapture before the coming Millennium, and so did my grandfather and uncles on my mother's side. My Uncle Charles on my mother's side engaged in debates on the topic with leaders of other churches, refuting those who believed in "a-millennialism" (the Millennium is figurative and is now in progress) and "post-millennialism" (Christ returns after the Millennium, not before it).

There was a lot of teaching about exactly who would be qualified for the Rapture and who would be left behind. The Church of Christ believed that Jesus is the "One Way" to God for everyone in the world, and we believed that we were the only ones truly following the "One Way." Thus, most people in my denomination thought that only Church of Christers would be able to go up in the Rapture. Even other Christians, such as Presbyterians, Methodists and Catholics—and possibly even Baptists—were probably destined to face the "Tribulation," a time of extreme suffering that is prophesied to come on the earth after the Rapture. During this Tribulation the Anti-Christ would rule the Earth, and enormous corruption and evil would be rampant throughout all nations. Preparing for Rapture was a way to escape the horrors of the Tribulation, and we wanted to be sure we were ready. The hope of Rapture was also motivation for evangelism. If we wanted other people to be saved from hell and tribulation, we needed to convert them to the true path.

We believed that the Rapture of the saints was imminent—it could happen any day. When we parted on the Lord's Day, one of the elders would often say, "We will meet again next Sunday, if the Lord tarries." We listened to fictional stories and tapes that depicted instances of people suddenly disappearing from the earth and leaving their puzzled friends and family behind to face the terrible "Tribulation." "What happened to Uncle Ted and Aunt Martha? And why am I still here?!" These stories were the forerunners of books such as the "Left Behind" series that has been wildly popular with some Christians today.

Resurrection also colored our view of contemporary news and politics, just as it colors it today for many conservative and evangelical Christians. We regarded the establishment of the state of Israel as the profound fulfillment of prophecy and expected that within one generation (forty years) of its founding the "end times" would come and the Rapture would occur, followed by the Tribulation. Many church writers found signs of the end everywhere, interpreting current events and technological innovations as fulfillment of prophecy. One of the popular writers was Hal Lindsey, who wrote *The Late Great Planet Earth*. These interpreters of prophecy were the forerunners of televangelists who preach similar doctrines today.

During my youth, there was a lot of speculation about who would be the anti-Christ, the powerful figure who will be the embodiment of the Devil and lead the world into Armageddon. At one time everyone I knew earnestly believed it was Henry Kissinger, because he was doing so much negotiation around the time of the 6-Day War in Israel. Many people watched the development of the European Union, believing that as soon as there were ten nations in it the Anti-Christ would come, the Rapture would occur, and the Tribulation would begin. There are now more than ten nations in the EU, and our modern apocalypse watchers have duly adapted their interpretation of the signs. Even though Jesus said no one knows the "day and the hour," many deem it expedient to read the "signs of the times."

The hope of Rapture was a strong motivating factor to live a godly life in service to others so that we could rise up with Christ in the midst of our usual daily activities. Since we didn't know when the event would occur, we needed to be ready at any moment. We performed service with our heavenly hope in mind, but we also minded the truth of our hearts, trying to make sure that they were in tune with the will of God.

The belief in resurrection had powerful effects on me. It ingrained in me the conviction that the current circumstances, no matter how they may appear, are not the final indicator of reality. There is a greater, more powerful reality which says that righteousness will be rewarded and that the reward is deliverance from the sorrow, death, tribulation, and evil that are in this world. A positive result of this for me was that it motivated me to live a life of faith and service with a pure heart toward God. A less positive result was that I had the impression God will give the righteous ones a ticket out of suffering; therefore, if one suffers very much, it is because she is not righteous enough and does not have enough faith. Later in life, as I suffered with chronic, crippling illness, this assumption would contribute to my feeling that God had abandoned me, a feeling with which I would struggle for many years.

Even though our teaching on Resurrection was extremely detailed, there were significant gaps. Jesus' powerful words, "I AM the Resurrection and the Life" only had meaning for eternity, holding the promise that if we believe in him and accept him as our Savior, we will go to heaven when we die. We did not apply them to overcoming the challenges and suffering of this present life. It was not until I was an adult and had been crippled for many years that I began to conceive of Christ's power of Rising as being available here and now, giving power and wholeness in this present life as well as the next.

The "One Way" teaching that undergirded the fundamentalist resurrection theology also had both positive and negative effects. It kept me focused on Christ and gave me strength for living a good life. At the same time, it also ingrained in me a hidden but powerful assumption that there is a narrow range of appropriate options available for any particular situation and that one must employ only those that directly square with one's own faith and culture. There was an underlying fear that experimenting outside that arena was not only dangerous but could actually result in intense suffering and going to hell. Later in life, this belief and fear kept me from exploring possibilities for healing outside my own familiar framework. Even more, it kept me from believing that God's grace is available everywhere at all times and that it can come to me abundantly and powerfully in ways I may not anticipate and through people and events that are surprising and possibly even strange. Perhaps these are some of the reasons why my healing was such a long time in coming.

When I think back on my experience of God when growing up, I am thankful for many things. I was surrounded by godly, loving people for whom worshiping and serving God was the center of their lives. Their reverence for scripture stimulated me to grow up knowing and loving the Bible, a legacy for which I am deeply grateful long after I have left behind some of the interpretations attached to it in my youth. Because I had such godly family members and such a strong church environment around me, I grew up loving God with all my heart and desiring to serve God with all my body, mind and strength, a heritage that is still the core of my life today.

Even with my thankfulness, I also know there were drawbacks to my fundamentalist youth. I remember lying awake at night as a young girl, looking out the small French windows over the moonlit bluff behind our farmhouse and telling God how much I wanted to serve him. I was very sad I couldn't be a preacher or missionary because I was a female. I seriously questioned God about why he made me a girl and not a boy. It was something I couldn't help, an innate flaw that seemed an unconquerable obstacle to my serving God in the way my heart desired.

My church's belief that everyone except us Church of Christers was destined for hell taught me to build walls, not bridges. I didn't know how to relate to people who had a faith and practice that was different from my own. These beliefs not only shut me off from many wonderful, godly people but also closed off my options for service because I couldn't search among other Christian communities for ministry that would fit my calling. I knew that Catholic women could become nuns, but I was sad that there was no opportunity for someone like me to enter such service. I had a heart for God but no way to express it except in the traditional ways that were modeled by those in my immediate context. Fortunately, I had many loving, godly, joyful women around me. Their examples guided me through the many years before the walls would come down and I would explore the larger world outside.

Falling Down

Dorothy in Kansas

I was on a bus, hurtling through the empty black space of central Kansas. It was so dark that when I looked out the window the sky was full of stars, and I could see meteors falling, falling, in every part of the sky. It seemed the sky was weeping. Strange things happen to people in Kansas. Little girls are suddenly swept up by tornados into strange places of tin men, scarecrows and cowardly lions. They venture over strange roads, confront wicked witches and have fantastic adventures, all the time desperately seeking the one who is running the Universe, hoping that when he is found everything will be made right. Strange things can happen in Kansas. A strange thing happened to me.

Harding College in Searcy, Arkansas, was the same Church of Christ school that my mother, aunts, uncles and sister attended—it was the family thing to do. It was also the college that produced most of the pastors and revival preachers for Churches of Christ. I was excited about going there because I thought it would be a little bit like heaven, with only godly, righteous people who were living godly, righteous lives and doing godly, righteous things day in and day out. From my earliest memory I had wanted to be a minister or missionary, but, since my denomination did not allow women to hold any position of leadership in the church, I decided to be an English and speech teacher instead, a profession that was safely within in the boundaries of my faith and practice.

Rules were strict at Harding in order to guard the morals of the students and perpetuate solid values for the future generations. At that time (it's different now) women had to wear skirts and dresses all the time except for sporting events, when only long pants were allowed. Women were not allowed to go off campus without sign-out permission from the Dean of Women Students. On hayrides, there was a law that hay could be no deeper than three inches in order that males and females should not get too comfortable down there in the hay. There were a lot of jokes on campus about how strict the rules were—for example, that girls should not wear patent leather shoes because they reflect up. Polk-a-dot dresses were in disrepute because they invited lustful ideas by guys who might want to poke the dots. I wore patent leather shoes, but I checked the reflectivity and felt it was in an acceptable range. I eschewed polk-a-dots.

Women had a ten o'clock curfew that was announced by the ringing of the campus bell. Guys, however, could stay out later and go off campus without permission, an inequality that was no doubt due to the theological superiority of males. Alcoholic beverages were, of course, strictly forbidden, although even that blindfolded administration must have known that "boys will be boys" and surely must have heard a few of the wild tales about after hours shenanigans.

Dancing was regarded as sinful, so social club "fetes" were usually formal dinners with some kind of entertainment program. There was a strict rule against guys putting their arms around girls, and such an infraction occurring in the little white swings on campus could be reprimanded by a passing faculty member. Brother Benson, the college President once announced in chapel that he had been walking across campus and had seen what seemed to be a "snake" curling around a young woman's shoulders in one of the swings. He looked over the top of his glasses and said in his southern drawl, "Young people, don't be snakey." The archetypal reference to the Garden of Eden connected sexuality strongly to our fallen natures, but, as with Adam and Eve, failed to deter snakey behavior when no one was watching.

Chapel attendance was mandatory every weekday, with only three misses allowed during a semester. A doctor's excuse was required for illness. Attendance at Sunday worship at the College Church was *de rigueur*. If one did not attend, it was an indication of "backsliding," a condition that could negatively affect one's social status. The campus was all white racially, which was typical of all the Churches of Christ I knew about. But it was the early 60's, and the racial issues were heating up more and more after riots in Little Rock. While I was at Harding, the first three black students were admitted to the school, with serious ceremony and prayer. Most people I knew thought Martin Luther King was a Communist, a designation only slightly better than the Antichrist. I didn't find out until I was a student there for a while that the college was at least a sympathizer, if not a sponsor, of the extreme right wing John Birch Society. I wasn't politically astute.

I was very happy at Harding College, to begin with. I auditioned and got into the A Cappella, the premier choir on campus. I went on some tours with them, mostly visiting other churches of Christ around the country. I loved music and singing, and the choir was a wonderful experience of fellowship and fun.

Between my freshman and sophomore years, I joined a mission group, raised funds for myself and went on a mission trip to a ghetto area in Glasgow, Scotland. This was an expression of my deep desire to share the gospel with others and an attempt to satisfy my innate but frustrated calling to ministry. Evangelism was an activity allowed to women as long as we had no leading role in public worship and confined our teaching to women and children.

The reason I was on the bus in Kansas was that I became active in the campus drama group. I gravitated toward it because I really liked drama and because I was headed toward the English/Speech degree. I soon found that the drama people, even at a "righteous" place like this college, were a little bit offbeat, a little bit liberal, a little bit more loose than others on campus in spirit, dress, and actions. Even so, I found that I liked them. Their creativity tended to push them toward the boundaries of what was accepted in that particular framework, and they challenged me to think about my own values and how I wanted to express them. My association with them tended to put me in the somewhat more "weird" category on campus, even though by the standards of any other college, our group was virginal. I wore heavier makeup than some other girls on campus, which felt comfortable because of the theatre connection. I was a friendly person, often saying a cheery "Hello!" to other students on the sidewalks. I discovered, however that I was regarded as "fake" for doing so. As I associated

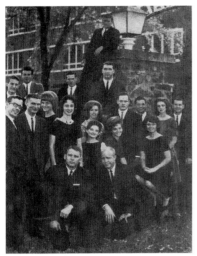
My first MS attack occurred while I was on a college drama tour in 1965.

with drama folks more, I began to feel that the outward social righteousness on campus was hypocritical and restrictive.

Our drama troupe made several tours of the Third and Fifth Armies, performing in army dining halls, theatres and clubs, as well as at the prison in Fort Leavenworth, Kansas. Touring was hard, exhausting work, setting up and tearing down, traveling long hours by bus. It threw all of us in the troupe together for good times and bad times, working, playing, sleeping—it was a social pressure cooker. Everyone's feelings, thoughts and problems came out into the open. Marnie was from a broken home. Norm was secretly gay. Nathan hid his agnosticism under a veil of piety to retain his campus popularity. I was deeply involved in everyone's emotions and relationships. I also fell head over heels in love with Tom Raynard, a senior member of the troupe. He did not return my affection.

By the end of my third drama trip, in the middle of my sophomore year, stress was taking a toll on me. At an evening performance in a large army theatre in Colorado, I misjudged a step in the dark and plunged over the edge of the stage, seriously bruising myself. As I nursed my wounds, I wondered how I happened to make such a silly mistake. The next day the tour was over and we headed home.

So there we were, riding through the night in the frozen cornfields of Kansas, without a sign of light or life anywhere for miles around. I shifted my position to get more comfortable in my seat, and a lightning bolt shot through my body. I grabbed the seat in front of me, gasping for breath. I thought, "Is lightning striking our bus?" I look outside, but there was no storm. The sky was still clear and raining only stars. I looked around at my friends in nearby seats, and they were sleeping quietly, worn out from the long drama tour, trying to catch all the shut-eye they could during the most boring part of our long trip home. I leaned back in the seat and rested my head against my pillowed coat. My body seemed heavy, as though I was weary from living a hundred years. I moved my right arm and it tingled like it had gone to sleep. "That's funny," I thought. "I wasn't even lying on it." The bus passed over a portion of highway that was under construction, crunching through gravel and hitting potholes that rattled the frame of our old bus. My body cringed as electric shocks ran through my arms and legs again. Oddly, I don't recall feeling fear. I didn't have anything in my experience to tell me I should be afraid. I knew nothing about the feelings I was having or what they meant. It was pure pain and pure amazement. All I could think of was, "What is happening here? Something is very wrong."

The bus came to a halt at one of those nondescript all-night truck stops that barely broke the monotony of long trips through nowhere in the days before all-service BP stations with McDonald's inside. Back in those good ol' days, it was always the same—chips, soda and an outdoor-access restroom with pee on the seat. I started down the aisle of the bus and found myself grasping the seats for stability. My feet didn't seem to anticipate where my body was going, and I felt like I might do a fast forward directly on my face. I clutched the folding-door handles of the bus as I dizzily placed my feet on the steps, then stepped down and down again, gripping my coat around me against the bitter cold. I headed unsteadily for the door of the truck stop. Inside, I bought some chips, but when I tried to eat them, my stomach roiled. I went outside and waited my turn for the washroom, all the while leaning against the door for support. I kept my eyes closed so my friends wouldn't see them rolling in my head. I didn't want them to think I had gone off my rocker. When my turn came, I went in and cleared the toilet seat with shaky hands, carefully putting paper on the sides and back. Loosening my clothes seemed to take a long time, and for some reason the buttons and zipper seemed to resist my clumsy fingers. As I lowered myself to the stool, another lightning bolt charged through my body, and I fell the rest of the way, hitting the sides of the stall. My torso flopped over crazily. I sat there with my head down, wondering how I would get out of the restroom with my clothes on. I rested for a little bit, thinking those outside waiting would be getting upset about my long stay. Finally, I gathered my strength, clumsily pulled my clothes back on and staggered out into the cold and back onto the bus. Since everyone was in a sleepy haze, they didn't seem to notice there was anything wrong with me. I curled up in my seat and closed my eyes, hoping it would all go away. Stars exploded all night long in my body. My personal sky was falling. Strange things happen in Kansas.

When the bus rolled into Searcy and back onto the campus, I thought maybe the universe would right itself, maybe the funnel cloud would reverse and land me back on terra firma in my own familiar room, in my own familiar skin. But that didn't happen. I put a brave front on for the world, but the fragile interior collapsed when I was checking my mail in the student center. Another blitz went through my body, and I staggered backward against the wall. Some fellow students looked up in alarm and asked what was wrong. "Nothing, nothing," I said, but I knew it was something, something very bad.

I took myself over to the campus clinic, and the doctors immediately put me in the hospital for testing. The lightning blitzes through my nervous system continued, as well as extreme sensitivity and electrical sensations on my skin. Doctors checked me for myasthenia gravis and other ailments, but could not reach any conclusions. In those days there were no MRI's to scan the brain and nervous system for abnormalities. My friends came to see me, and I put on a brave, happy show while they were there, only to collapse as soon as they went out the door.

Finally, I called my parents. "I'm not doing so well, Daddy," I said.

"Well, what's the matter, Susie?" That was a pet name from childhood that he used for special, tender times. His voice was worried.

"I don't know. When I try to stand up, I have these terrible pains. I'm in the hospital now. Sometimes I feel okay, but then afterward I feel really bad."

"What do the doctors say?"

"They don't know, Daddy. No one seems to know."

"Do we need to come and get you? We'll do that if we need to."

I was embarrassed about causing so much trouble. It was a 450-mile trip. "I really hate to make you come all that way. Maybe if we just wait, the problem will go away."

"Don't you worry about that. Let me talk to the doctor. If we need to come, we'll come right away."

The doctors were stumped. They had no assurance to offer my parents and suggested it was a good idea to come and get me. My parents made the long trip the next day. I said a tearful farewell to my friends, and Mother and Daddy bundled me into the old blue Chevy, propped me up with pillows and drove me home.

For the whole spring semester I rested at the farm, taking weekly art lessons and helping out occasionally in my father's real estate office. The peace and quiet of home and the beloved fields and forests gradually calmed me and healed me of a broken heart, broken spirit and broken body.

Strange things happen in Kansas. I did not know until years later that as I traveled the dark road on that bus I had my first attack of multiple sclerosis. Like Dorothy, who was picked up by a tornado and swept to a strange land, that event would eventually propel me into a life as strange and confusing as OZ.

Signs in the Heavens, Signs in Earth

The phone rang, and when I answered, my mother said, "Anna Sue?" She always called me by both of my given names. I could tell by her voice she had something special on her mind.

"Hi Mother, how's camp?" The Church of Christ rented Camp Krietenstein from the Boy Scouts for a couple of weeks each summer, and she was the women's counselor. I had attended the same camp for several years as a high schooler and had fond memories of it.

"It's good," she said warmly. "I have a bunch of great girls, and we're learning songs and having a great time. Do you think you might come up to visit?"

I was in summer school, trying to make up for the time I lost at college when my body blew up. I was feeling normal by now, but I hadn't really intended to go to the camp. "Oh, I don't know. Is there anyone there that I know?"

"Well, as a matter of fact . . ." She lowered her tone of voice and said rather intimately, "Yes, there is someone here. Do you remember Don York?"

My heart skipped a beat. Of course I remembered Don York. He was on the Scout staff and pretty much ran the place. He was a big husky football and rugby player, strong as an ox, able to heave canoes on and off trucks with scarcely a thought. We had exchanged coy glances for a couple of summers while I was at camp, and then, the summer after my senior year in high school, his interest perked up. We had actually even held hands, which was a pretty far out thing to do in that strict environment with all the preachers looking on. He had just finished a year studying physics at MIT, a place I had never heard of but had the impression was a pretty tough school out East somewhere. I wasn't very sophisticated about such things. After I started college, we exchanged a few letters, but time and distance was not in our favor. I fell in love with a preacher boy from Montgomery, Alabama, then fell out of love, then got involved with the drama group. We lost contact.

"Don York?" I said. "Yes, I remember him. "Is he still around?"

"Oh, yes, he certainly is!" Mother said with a twinkle. Then she grew a little wistful. "You know what he did last night?"

"No, what?"

"Well, after the evening program was over, we were walking back to the dining hall, and there he was beside me. We started talking, and I said how beautiful the sky was. He said, 'Would you like to go look at some stars?' Well, of course I said yes. Then we went out into the middle of the playing field, and it was really dark, and you could see all the stars and the Milky Way, bright and clear. He pointed out Leo, Lyra and the Big Dipper—he seemed to know them all. He really loves astronomy. Then, you know what he did?"

"What?" I asked.

"Well, he waved his arm across the sky, and he said, "It's all mine." Her voice was full of wonder and admiration.

"Really," I said.

"Mmhmm."

"Well, maybe I'll drive up there this evening."

Don may have had my mother's head in the stars, but his work at the camp was less than celestial. On the evening I arrived, we sighted each other as he was washing garbage cans behind the dining hall. He had a hose in one hand and a garbage can lid in the other. As I stepped out the back door of the mess hall, he looked up, then looked down at himself, then looked up again. With a twinkle and laugh, he said warmly, "It's good to see you." I laughed too, appreciating his predicament and the anti-romantic humor of the situation. Somehow it felt comfortable and good, and it seemed like life changed right there in front of the garbage cans. Bells rang (the dinner bell), and a choir sang (campers singing "We are table number one, where is table two"). We definitely made a cosmic connection.

After he cleaned up, we took a walk by the lake and talked for hours. He showed me the stars that were shooting across the sky in the annual Perseide meteor shower, and I was even more entranced than

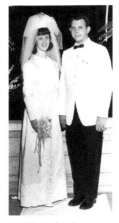
Life looks bright on our wedding day in 1966.

my mother. I felt this was someone I could trust with my own personal stars. That night he broke up with the girl he had dated for five years, and two days later he asked me to marry him. He was not one to fool around once he made up his mind!

We married the following June after his graduation from MIT and moved to Yerkes Observatory in Williams Bay, Wisconsin, where Don would study for a Ph.D. in astronomy from the University of Chicago. Ours was a marriage that started with stars in our eyes and continued through all the years, literally, with a focus on heaven.

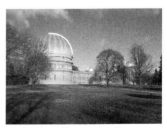
Yerkes Observatory houses the largest refracting telescope in the world.

We started life in a two-room cabin with a wood-fired stove and an outdoor john down the sidewalk—that's the honest truth! For a bath we had to go fifty yards down the sidewalk to the "big house" where our Norwegian landlords lived. One of my favorite stories is about the night I got locked in the outhouse at midnight at ten below zero with twelve inches of snow on the ground. Don was asleep inside the cottage and couldn't hear my yells, so I thought I was done for. Searching in the dark, I discovered that there actually was a real Sears catalogue in there. I tore a piece off of the cover, stuck it through the crack in the door, shivering all the while,

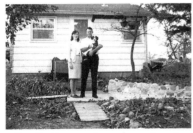
Our first home, a two-room cottage in Williams Bay, Wisconsin.

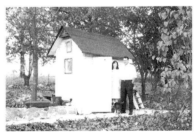
Our private, luxury outhouse, complete with Sears catalog!

and gently lifted the wood block that had accidentally dropped down to lock the door from the outside. When I got inside, I stuck my icy feet right in the middle of Don's back!

We were poor but didn't notice it—we had the American Dream in our sights. Our biggest financial splurge was on Friday nights when we shelled out a dollar fifty for all-you-can-eat fish fries in the little towns around the county. We saved our pennies in a sock all week for a scrumptious Saturday night ice cream treat at the Keg Room in beautiful "downtown" Williams Bay, a summer tourist village that rolled up the streets in winter. Don's favorite was double chocolate fudge, and mine was pistachio almond.

I finished my senior year at Beloit College, which was up the road thirty miles, and then began teaching at Big Foot High School, which was in the small town of Walworth not far from Yerkes. I always joked that I got my job there by showing my shoe size—a country girl size 11.

I was not only happy in my new marriage, but as a brand new, idealistic teacher, I was unstoppable. I designed and inaugurated a speech program for the school, directed school plays and led my drama club to take first place out of 450 schools in the state drama contest. I shook up the system by getting my speech classes involved in local politics. We raised community awareness and campaigned for a new school building program that was coming up for a vote. The referendum passed, and I was convinced it was at least partially due to our vigorous campaigning efforts.

One night I was onstage directing my students in a production of the original plays they had written, when suddenly, right in the middle of "Move a little farther downstage—" Boom! A severe pain flashed through my chest, doubling me over. One of my students said, "Hey, whoa! Are you okay?"

I grabbed my stomach and reached down as though tying my shoe. "Yeah, sure," I responded. No teacher wants to seem flakey in front of her students.

But I wasn't all right. The pains continued to recur at embarrassing times in front of my classes, and it took extra energy to hide it from them and from my teaching colleagues. My energy began to feel tenuous and fluttery. The stress seemed to be getting to me. I finally broke down and went to see Dr. Bender, the father of one of my sophomore students. I was a little concerned that he might let his son know I had come to see him, but in such a small town there weren't many choices. After EKGs and other tests, he told me he thought it was "just stress." He knew about all the activities I was promoting at school and told me I needed to slow down. That was pretty hard to understand since other people were doing a lot too. I couldn't understand what was different about me that stress should have such a bad effect.

I struggled through my classes and activities throughout the autumn of that year and hoped Don would soon finish his degree. He spent weeks plotting his observational data by pasting thousands of little black dots on white cardboard, representing the lines in stellar spectra. It was the days before computer graphics. By the time he graduated from the University of Chicago in the middle of my third teaching year, I was feeling weak and in serious need of a rest. My body was giving me signs of another coming disaster. We packed all our belongings in a U-Haul trailer and headed East.

Moving Out in Spirit

The *Copernicus* space telescope satellite was the first big successful telescope that was launched into space. When Don finished his Ph.D. at the University of Chicago, he got a job working on the *Copernicus* project for Princeton University. The satellite was being built at NASA headquarters in Greenbelt, Maryland, so we moved to the Washington D.C. area. We settled into a little house in the country across from the Bottners, a big family with a huge garden and a bountiful harvest that they freely shared with us. I have fond memories of sitting on Mom Bottner's porch shelling peas and husking corn. It was a time of quietness and healing in body, mind and spirit.

We had our first baby, Sean, in 1971, and I joyously entered into motherhood. We were active in our church, especially in ministering to teens, and we had lots of friends with whom we shared our life and faith. I was full of praise and thanksgiving for God's goodness. I remember very clearly a conversation I had with God one afternoon while driving home with the baby. I spoke to God and said, "Lord, life is just so good, I can't imagine how anything could be better."

Apparently God could imagine something better. A short time later, Billie, our minister's wife, gave me Pat Boone's book, *A New Song*. In this book the popular singer and actor described how he received the "baptism of the Holy Spirit," including speaking in tongues, and how it changed his life and his career. Since speaking in tongues and all such activities described in the book were taboo in our church, Billie must have thought I would find it a curiosity. In fact, the book changed my life forever. You see, Pat Boone was a Church of Christer, like me. His experience made me feel deeply joyous, and my heart began to yearn for a deeper, more experiential relationship with God. I thought if it could happen to Pat Boone, perhaps it could also happen to me.

Our church taught that the age of miracles was past. I began to search the scriptures diligently to see if it was really possible for people to have experiences such as speaking in tongues and physical healing in our day and age. The only materials I had on the subject were those put out by the Church of Christ, which made strong arguments against it. I used them to start my search. I got a New English version of the Bible and read it voraciously, looking carefully at every reference to the Spirit. The Holy Spirit began to leap from every page, speaking that God is real and present and that the Spirit is powerful and available in all its fullness right now, today. My heart began to swell with even greater love and I yearned passionately to be filled with the Spirit.

I began to believe that all the gifts of the Spirit are available now if only we "ask, seek and knock." I had opportunity to test this when Sean was about nine months old. It was late autumn, and all the babies at church were coming down with a terrible flu that caused high fevers and lasted for a couple of weeks. Sean got this flu, and he was extremely ill. None of us got any sleep at night. I gave him baths and baby aspirin, but it seemed to make no difference. On about the third day, I said, "Well, Lord, I know you are able to heal this baby, so in the name of Jesus I ask you to do it now." I anointed him with some oil, put on a fresh diaper and laid him in his crib. I turned and walked out the door and shut it, thanking the Lord for taking care of him.

Little baby Sean slept all night. In the morning I heard the crib rattling vigorously and went into his room to find him beaming a smile and announcing loudly that he wanted some breakfast. I joyously picked up him and hugged him, saying, "Oh, good morning, praise God, you're fine today, oh praise God!"

I knew with all my heart that Christ had healed him. My joy was overflowing. I went around the house singing, praising and thanking God. I also called my pastor's wife to share the news that Jesus had healed my baby.

"Billy, you'll never believe what has happened. You know how sick Sean has been?"

"Yes," she said. "How is he doing today?"

"He's fine! He's good! He's completely well!" I said.

"Oh, really? That's good to hear."

"Yes," I said, "Last night he was so terrible. He couldn't breathe, and his temperature was over 103 degrees. So I prayed for him and put some oil on him and asked Jesus to heal him. Then I put him in his crib and went out the door. He slept all night, and this morning he's fine. Jesus has healed my baby!"

I finished my story and waited for the joyous response. To my surprise, I met silence and a palpable skepticism at the other end of the phone line. She finally said, "Well, you know he probably wasn't actually healed. It was probably just a coincidence. Those things happen, you know." Her words were like ice water in my face. This was my pastor's wife speaking. I was astonished that someone could be so blind to such a wonderful event and not even willing to express thankfulness with me!

But that was only the beginning of my education about people's responses to unfamiliar spiritual experiences. I had been encouraging the teen girls in my Sunday school class to pray and expect God to answer. For example, the pastor's daughter had a headache one evening and I suggested she pray for it to go away. It did go away! I saw her eyes begin to light up in faith and love.

A few days later, Billie felt obliged to bring me the bad news connected with this joyful event. It seems she was once more inclined to deliver her message by phone instead of in person. "You know, Anna, you really need to be careful about what you are teaching our teens. They are so young and impressionable that they don't know what to believe. You have a responsibility to them. If you teach them these kinds of things, that they can pray and be healed, they may begin to think that's the way it is. We all know that the age of miracles is past. When they pray and God doesn't answer their prayers, they may lose their faith."

Shortly after that, I received yet another phone call from the director of the regional church camp who had signed me up as a camp counselor. "Anna, I know we approved your application to be a counselor, but it looks like we're not going to be able to have you fill that role."

I was shocked and disappointed. "Oh? Why is that?"

"Well, we've had someone call from your church with complaints about what you've been teaching the teens. I really have to take that into consideration."

"Well, I'm so surprised," I said. "We've been doing the youth ministry for quite a while. Could you tell me who you spoke to? Maybe I can clear it up."

"I'm afraid I can't tell you that. I'm sorry, but that's just the way it is now."

I hung up feeling confused and hurt. I had a suspicion about who had made the phone call. I tried to find out what was going on, but no one would answer my questions, and no one came to talk to me to address their concerns. Within a short time, the whole structure of the youth ministry in our church was changed, and Don and I, who had been at the center of it, were left completely out, without anyone giving us forewarning or explanation. I was also asked not to participate in the summer door-to-door evangelistic campaign. A well-meaning friend admonished me to "just be quiet about it." The protection impulse against heresy was very strong in our church. I was learning that growth in spirit can be perceived by those close to you as threatening and even dangerous. It can cause people not only to withdraw but also to react negatively and actively reject. And I wasn't even speaking in tongues—yet!

I continued my spiritual search. It gradually dawned on me that if what I read in scripture about the Spirit were true, it could not be contained in any one church or denomination. Nor could it be tied to any particular mode of worship or even to any set of doctrinal laws. After all, Jesus himself said, "The wind blows where it chooses, and you hear the sound of it, but you do not know where it comes from or where it goes. So it is with everyone who is born of the Spirit." It seemed this might mean that the Spirit could choose to be in any church and to empower all kinds of people, regardless of their denomination and the details of their beliefs. The Spirit that broke the barriers between

Jews and Gentiles could not be contained by human definitions or by established religious institutions. I realized that anyone—even Catholics!—could be Christians. Astonishingly, I now began to know, deep in my heart, that I had Christian brothers and sisters around the world in all denominations. The church walls, so strongly and solidly built up in my own religious upbringing and experience came tumbling down, just like Jericho's walls. From my point of view it was the Spirit that was doing the tumbling!

As the walls came down, I sought out a charismatic worship service at Truro Episcopal Church in a southwestern suburb of D.C. and convinced Don to accompany me there on a Saturday evening. It was the first time I crossed the boundary into another denomination, and I did it with butterflies in my stomach, feeling as though I were trespassing into dangerous and forbidden territory. Even so, I longed for the Spirit so much that I entered the church and soon began to feel the lovely warmth of the Spirit around me.

Truro was one of the bastions of the charismatic movement in the Washington area, and the worship was strange, joyous and wonderful. After a time of praise, thanksgiving and testimonies, the leader of the group said, "There's a stream of the Holy Spirit flowing just above our heads. If you just put up your hands, you can receive it." I had never raised my hands in worship in my life, but, as the group sang softly, my desire was so great that I slowly, tearfully put up both of them, completely oblivious to what my astonished husband would think. As my hands reached about the height of my head, I began to feel a warm, flowing stream, like spiritual water, flowing over me. As my hands went higher, the river began cascading down, around, in and through me in glorious warm waves, flowing, washing, cleansing, filling. It was the most exquisite sensation I have ever had in my life. When my arms came down, the river continued to flow, and I felt transported to a different dimension, cradled in a loving, warm sea of the Spirit. On the way home, still caressed in that warmth, I began to speak the first words of a language I had never known or learned.

The sensory experience of the Spirit went on for weeks, with varying intensity. Every time I praised God the river of warmth would flow in, around and through me, carrying me along in its stream. A particular phrase of the new language became very familiar. I had the impression that it sounded like French, even though I had never studied that language. Don had studied French, so I tried the phrase out on him. He said, "Oh yes, there's just one word I don't recognize. He looked it up in the Petite Larousse and then translated: "Thank you, Lord, for my new language (a particular French dialect)." From that moment Don knew there was something amazing happening.

There were times when I would pray and move from one language to another to another to another, having the sensation of moving without any barrier through time and space. I began to sing songs in the spirit and to write my own songs, which I accompanied on the guitar. I was full of praise day and night.

But I didn't know what to do next. I didn't know what the wonderful energy was that was flowing through me, I didn't understand the meaning of the experiences, and I didn't know how to develop the gifts or apply them to the circumstances of my life. I was afloat in the sea of the Spirit with no guide.

The first person with whom I came into contact was a Church of Christ man whom I would later describe as a "toe-dipper" in the Spirit. Joe liked to flirt with the charismatic experience, but he would not risk his position in his church to consider any serious changes in his life. It was the titillating aspects of the experience that seemed to attract him. I was young and inexperienced, and he was the only Church of Christ person I knew who knew anything about the Spirit. I naively trusted him.

Those were the times when flashy, charismatic televangelists such as Jim Bakker and Jimmy Swaggert were in their heyday—before they were exposed for fraud and adultery. I had never had any interest in them because my own background taught me to have a more reserved approach to worship, and they seemed shallow and flamboyant. Even so, they had a powerful effect on many people, giving the impression that being full of the Spirit was more about personal magnetism than holiness, more about reaping ego satisfaction than serving others.

One day when I was working on an assignment for a temp agency, Joe called and suggested we have lunch and some prayer time. Swept up by my new spiritual experience, I didn't anticipate that I was the dish he had in mind for lunch. When he laid hands on me to pray, I knew they were a little too humanly friendly to connect me with heaven. Deeply embarrassed and burning with anger and shame, I reported him to his elders and had nothing more to do with him. Don didn't tell me until years later that the charlatan called him on the phone at least three times, telling him that while we were praying I had tried to grab his penis! Don told him he was sick and needed to get help. I was grateful for a loving, trusting husband.

The experience was scary. It caused me to reflect on how it is possible for a person to have power but have no idea how to use it properly. It seemed I was sailing in dangerous seas. I had an experience but no one to interpret how I should respond or teach me how to progress. Not everyone was trustworthy. I needed someone with experience and wisdom to help me steer my ship.

I met Deje and Sissy while I was selling Bibles at a local book fair. They invited me to attend a prayer meeting, and I accepted. When I walked in the door, I heard a group singing "Heavenly Rivers," a song written by a member of the group. I felt like I was stepping once again into that heavenly river. As I let the music wash over me, I felt like I had come home. I settled into their prayer group and their local events and ministries, including regular visits with Deje and Sissy to the Glendale Hospital, a welfare hospital outside Washington, D.C. Don and I also began to attend the larger fellowship meetings, which were led by Ellen Blackwell, a gifted female teacher who had her roots in the early revival days of the Assembly of God.

Ellen had started her own interdenominational teaching ministry to address the needs of those coming into the charismatic experience with no preparation and knowledge of the Spirit. I had grown up in a denomination that did not allow women to have any leadership roles, and she was the first strong female teacher I had encountered. She knew more Bible than any of the men I had ever known, and, besides that, she was in tune with the Spirit that infused the book. She taught and practiced healing and other powerful gifts of the Spirit, but, at the same time, she was very strong on disciplines of holiness, prayer, fasting, and modest dress. Her teaching and style, which contrasted strongly with that of charismatic televangelists, appealed to my conservative upbringing. Since I had wanted to be a minister from the time I was a child, she became a role model for me, opening the spiritual meaning of scripture, giving it application, and nourishing my hungry soul. Even though the teaching was completely Bible-based and the disciplines were serious, I felt a freedom I had never known before. In this interdenominational group I was moving out into a larger world where people are tied together by spirit rather than by doctrine and tradition.

I Feared a Fear

As Deje, Sissy and I entered the door of Glendale Hospital, the smell of antiseptic assaulted our senses. It was almost palpable, so strong that you knew that the underlying smells required industrial-strength sanitation. The lighting in the hallway was dim, flickering dully off slick green walls. The heavy paint was chipped here and there and clumsily re-patched. It was a county hospital. Funds were low for running a facility for long-term residents who could not pay. All of the residents were on welfare and many had been abandoned to that smelly, steamy backwater of humanity because their relatives could not or did not want to deal with their illness. Many had multiple sclerosis or other crippling, disfiguring diseases. Blind, deformed, and helpless, they had little hope of ever leaving this place.

We headed toward the second floor balcony, passing inmates who had been wheeled into the hall while their rooms were being mopped. Distorted faces and blank, rheumy eyes silently groaned the stories of their tragic pasts and the horror of endless empty days. As we went through an area with beds in a larger, open space, Deje said softly, "Over there is a woman who has no face." I looked in that direction and saw a woman with a pulpy mass on the front of her head. There were no eyes, and there was a hole where the mouth would usually have been. Her face had been eaten away by cancer. I swallowed hard and looked quickly away. The image would haunt me long into the future.

When we arrived at Cora's place on the balcony, she was sitting quietly in her wheelchair in a worn, red-checked cotton robe. She had multiple sclerosis. It was my first personal encounter with someone who had the disease. Her limp feet, which were resting on the foot flaps of the chair, were stuck into clean but threadbare pink slippers. Coal black hair accentuated the paleness of her features. Her light blue eyes searched sightlessly toward the sound of visitors. The disease had stolen her vision.

It was a hot day. The windows were open and a ceiling fan churned slowly over our heads, barely stirring the heavy, torpid air. Deje and Sissy greeted Cora warmly, taking her hand tenderly, kissing her on the cheek and stroking her shoulder. They came regularly to help her and a few other women with small tasks and personal hygiene, such as washing and curling hair. They brought inspirational tapes and reading materials and did an occasional devotional with songs and Bible readings. I walked the halls with them, prayed with various people, heard their stories, and helped them in small ways. I thought those with multiple sclerosis were the most pitiful human beings I had ever seen.

I only went to the Glendale hospital a few times. Each time, when I exited into the sunshine, I felt I needed to purge the horror by taking deep gulps of fresh, clean air. I would look around at the green trees and blue sky, thanking God for life and health and for people who loved me. I would walk down the sidewalk, thinking to myself, "I am walking away from here, but they are staying. They have nowhere else to go. They will be here till the day they die." I could not imagine a worse future than that. I recall saying to God, "Of all the things that could happen to me, please, Lord, don't let it be multiple sclerosis!"

The Price of Liberty

It wasn't long after my new experience in the Spirit that Don and I permanently left the Church of Christ, the denomination that had been my family church and had nurtured me from birth. It was a painful departure, even though we left with a strong sense of hope and empowerment. We were experiencing that there is a price for new growth and liberty that is paid in the loss of familiar relationships and comfortable patterns of lifestyle. Change has its benefits, but it also has its costs. At this time of our lives, when we were young, strong and flexible, we thought the benefits were worth the price.

My family also learned the price of change. When I began to experience life in the Spirit, I decided I needed to tell my family about it, not knowing whether they would accept my testimony or decide to "excommunicate" me. While visiting them in Indiana, I shared my story with my parents and older sister, and they listened attentively. Then, after I left, they talked among themselves and decided that God might be opening a new understanding for them. In order to find out, they would just have to "go direct" and ask God themselves! They had a prayer meeting that lasted about five hours, seeking God with all their hearts. During that time, my mother saw a bright light, my father had a vision of Christ's heart, and my sister spoke in tongues!

This experience marked the beginning of an amazing renewal for all of them. My mother, who was already a spiritual dynamo, became even more of a powerhouse, reaching out to touch and heal anyone who came into her sphere. It was during this time that Mother began a nursery school, a prison ministry, and a nursing home ministry. Her compassion found tangible expression everywhere she turned.

My father's vision of Christ's heart strengthened him to receive healing from his own heart trouble. He threw away his nitro tablets and began once again to walk the hills and fields selling real estate. His office door was open to the community. Owners of businesses and farms around the area came there for advice and help in selling their property, and the local street people and handicapped stopped by for a rest and a short chat. He was active in local and county politics. He gave up reading his beloved Zane Grey westerns and began to devour scripture, especially books on the Second Coming of Christ. The turnaround in his own health gave him courage to believe God could do miracles for other people. He began to pray in church with such love and faith and with such tenderness of heart that people began to notice a change in him. The problems came when people discovered he actually expected answers!

My father had been an elder in the church for twenty years. Jerry and Wade, the other elders, finally came to him. "Ariel, we're concerned about you praying the way you're doing. It sounds like you actually expect these prayers to be answered. You know, Ariel, the miracles passed away when the apostles died. It's not according to good doctrine to be praying in that way. It sets a bad example for people. They will begin to expect things that aren't going to happen. We want you to stop praying that way."

My father told them his story of healing, his joy radiating from his face. "I have to do what my heart tells me," he said. "I don't feel I can just quench what the Spirit is doing."

Jerry and Wade were unimpressed. "Ariel, if you continue this way, we don't feel you are suitable to be an elder here." I'm sure they didn't realize they were speaking to the man who held the warranty deed to the church property!

Mother and Daddy prayed about what they should do. The Church of Christ had been the family church for generations. To leave it would be a blow not only to the church but also to their relationships in the extended family. But to stay would quench the life of the Spirit that was growing daily in them, and this they were not willing to do. One Sunday morning they went to the front of the church and read a scripture from the first chapter of I Corinthians. That scripture said that God's people would not lack any gift (including miracles) while waiting for the return of Christ. They said farewell and asked

God to bless the congregation; then they joined hands and walked down the aisle and out the church door forever. They never looked back and never took action on their rights to the deed.

During the next few years all of us had various experiences with the Holy Spirit and with people who were trying to live by the Spirit. There were wonderful answers to prayer, including healing, and there was an amazing flow of creativity in original songs, worship and other expressions. It was a rich time of faith and growth. Nevertheless, there was a mysterious element of uncertainty in all of it. There were manifestations we did not understand and could not control. Once we were all praying in a circle, and Ron Kizer just fell right over on the floor. We knew he wasn't sick, and we knew things like that sometimes happen, so we just kept praying and then sang a praise chorus. Ron had "fallen in the spirit." After a time, he got up from the floor and joined in the worship again. On more than one occasion I also fell in the spirit. It was like falling into a soft, cumulus cloud. Afterwards I would experience a boost in my spiritual commitment, but I don't know how other people felt after falling. A friend of mine once fell straight backward, like a falling tree, and hit her head on a wooden pew. She didn't feel it and later had no bruises or discomfort of any kind. She also said she felt like she was falling on a cloud. During big meetings in which a lot of people might be expected to fall, there were "catchers" to protect them on the way down.

Other strange things might happen too, such as laughing or even barking in the spirit. We concluded, "Well, that's the way the spirit moves." The Spirit seemed unpredictable. Even the charismatic healers in various meetings did not always seem to know what or how something would happen. There seemed to be certain circumstances of prayer, faith and worship that made a situation conducive to the "flow of the Spirit." Also, certain types of physical movements and certain types of sounds were characteristic, but they varied, depending on the specific culture of the group. In some groups there was a lot of shouting and jumping up and down, but other groups were quiet and liturgical. The Holy Spirit seemed to "work" in almost any type of religious setting. Even so, prayers were often prayed and attempts at healing were often made that had no discernible results.

We had moved out of the safe world of fundamentalist doctrine, away from black and white answers and clear-cut interpretations of a single denomination into a larger sphere in which the spirit moves like the wind and we do not know where it comes from and where it goes. Prayers could be answered or not, people could be healed or not, all because of God's "mysterious will." As we wrestled with these issues, none of us knew that soon I would be struck, for no apparent reason, with a horrible, incurable disease, a disease that would test our faith to the core, a disease that would seem to make me a victim of that inscrutable, divine will. I would long with all my heart for an altar call healing that would wipe out my disease forever. I would pray for it and seek it, but it would not come. I would seek the Spirit, but the Spirit would not answer my call.

Doing, Doing, Doing Too Much

The Tudor house had a large entryway, big enough to serve as a dining room, and assembled around the table was a motley crew of family, household residents, random friends and students who happened to drop in for supper, dessert or just to hang out. Don was at the far end with two-year-old Jeremy on a booster chair next to him. Jeremy had just spilled his milk for the second time. On the other side of him was Chandler, age three, who was being admonished to eat his "trees" (broccoli) by Rachel, a live-in who was recovering from drug and alcohol usage. She was a "PK" (preacher's kid) gone awry, and I thought I could help her out. Next to her was Jeff, a live-in student from Westminster Choir College and a card carrying schizophrenic. I had taken him on as a rehab case because he was from our church and needed someone. I was his someone. Sean, our 10-year-old, was asking for some tea, and Maurice, our four-year-old, was wondering when the birthday cake was coming. Don got up to pour tea in Sean's glass, and when he poured it, the stream missed the glass and went all over the table. He had just injured his eye playing squash, and the lack of binocular vision made him miss the target. Everyone around the table gave a whoop and did the "Wave," trying to escape the cascading liquid. The tea ran off the plastic table cloth onto an industrial-strength red carpet that was capable of digesting prodigious amounts of food and drink without looking at all the worse for wear. Just about that time, Fred and Janet, graduate students at Princeton, knocked on the door. It was Fred's birthday, and they were coming over for some cake and ice cream. I mopped the table, reassembled the troops, and pulled up two more chairs. When everyone was finished eating, we cleared the table and doused the lights so we could bring out the lighted cake. I had made it and decorated it myself, applying pastel blossoms, green sugar foliage and script lettering. I carried the lighted cake through door, accompanied by loud strains of "Happy Birthday to You." I looked around at the glowing faces. Just another night in the York household.

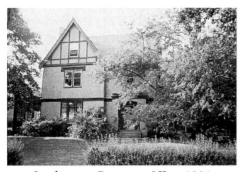
Our house in Princeton, NJ, in 1981.

Don and I had moved to Princeton, New Jersey, after *Copernicus*, the first space telescope, was successfully launched into space from Cape Canaveral. The next phase of his career would be spent at Princeton University, analyzing the data and writing research papers on the findings. Our first home in Princeton was a little two-bedroom cottage, but each time we added a child we moved to a larger home. Next it was a four-bedroom townhouse, and then the six-bedroom Tudor. We had three children in four years, two by C-section. While other women in Princeton were juggling careers, I was juggling babies.

True to my usual form, I was a dynamo. My faith was aflame, and it seemed to give me boundless energy. Some people even thought I was a kind of Wonder Woman, and, once I recovered physically from all the birthing, I had that image of myself as well. As I moved into maturity, I became more like my mother. I was one of those women who could keep six balls in the air at the same time I changed a diaper, cooked dinner, mopped the floor, and entertained guests. The big Tudor house was only three blocks from the Princeton University campus. We kept open house for the students in a Christian group there, often having two or three of them living with us, trying to rehab their lives after some psychological or academic trauma. I was counselor, confessor, and birthday-cake maker for them all. I loved it. I also made all my own clothes and more or less kept the house.

It was during this time that the pastor of our church opened a ministry of teaching for me. It was a Wednesday night class that started with about 15 people, both male and female. Within a year it had grown to more than 80 in attendance. We moved the class into the main sanctuary and added microphones, taping equipment and other support. It seemed that God was not only blessing me with a bountiful home and family life but was also answering my long-held desire to be a minister.

Between cake batter and diapers at home, I counseled and nourished bleeding souls who landed on my doorstep as a result of my classes. I believed that nobody's problems were too big for God and that I could help solve those problems. For example, there was Sherry, who was once the girlfriend of a famous mobster's son—this is true—I'm not making it up! She told me stories of flying all over the country with him and of watching while the "family" mapped out the takeover of a small country in Africa. She eventually became a Christian, and the turnaround in her life was so astonishing that several of her family members and friends also became Christians. Then, to top it all off, she inherited a million dollars from a rich uncle—cross my heart, it's the truth!

Sherry was only one of numerous high-intensity ministry situations. The roster of people living in our house was constantly changing. For example, there was the schizophrenic named Jeff. One day he had to be forcibly removed from the Westminster Choir College lunchroom when he announced publicly that he wanted to be castrated. Another day I got a call from Jutta, a white-haired, seventy-year-old German widow who had stayed in our house for a couple of weeks while her apartment was being repaired. She said, in her German brogue, "Anna, you have got to do something about Jeff. Do you know what he did today?"

I braced myself and said, "No, what did he do?"

"Well, he called me on the phone and told me he loved me and asked to marry me!"

"Oh, my!"

"Anna, he's crazy! The very idea, asking to marry me!" I agreed it would not be a good match and called his parents to come and get him.

Others had serious problems, but at least they did have all their marbles. Donna, a student who lived with us for several months, was struggling psychologically and spiritually with abuse by a stepfather.

Maria was an extreme insomniac whose insomnia ended when she spent her first night in our home. Lisa was a student on the verge of dropping out of school and being admitted to a mental institution. She moved into an upstairs room, and we organized her friends as an around-the-clock study and escort team to help her get through final exams and graduate on time.

In addition to the in-home ministry, there were numerous "out-patients" such as Peaches, a Japanese woman whose mother had been involved in voodoo when she was a child. Peaches would suddenly, uncontrollably erupt in strange sounds right in the middle of worship. Some of us got together and invited her to come for prayer to be delivered from a "bad spirit." She came gladly, and we prayed for her loudly and aggressively, demanding the spirit to depart. "In the name of Jesus! In the name of Jesus!" we shouted. As we did so, she described how the "pain" was moving in different parts of her body. We directed our hands toward the pain in karate-chop type movements until finally, with a shout, she was freed. She threw her hands up in the air and urinated on my red couch. I must confess that I hadn't counted on that particular response. I quietly cleaned it up, and we tended her lovingly. After she recovered for a few minutes, she fixed us some lunch, praising God all the while. She never manifested the problem again.

Life was very, very busy, and with the constant parade of unusual people through our home, it was certainly never boring! I thought life was very, very good. I felt like God was fulfilling my dream to do ministry, and I could see powerful evidence that God was at work in the people around me. I didn't know that all the childbirths, the care of the family, and the busy, stressful lifestyle were overloading my physical system. After I ministered to people, I didn't know how to protect myself by clearing out the emotional, psychological, and spiritual burdens of those to whom I was ministering. I was carrying the weight of the world on my shoulders and thought that was what

God wanted me to do. I didn't know that my propensity for doing too much was taking me headlong toward burnout. What I did discover, in early 1981, was that I was pregnant with our fifth child.

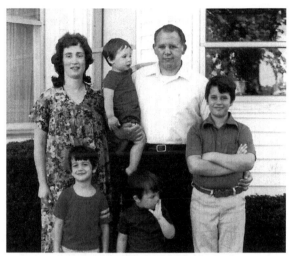

In 1981, I am pregnant and exhausted from bearing four children in five years.

Our Little Girl Dies

There are some events that are so profound you cannot speak of them for many years—and perhaps never at all. They become buried deep in the psyche, deep in the spirit, and they form our most fundamental thinking, feeling, and behavior. They create the warp and woof on which we weave the tapestry of our lives, but, like those deeply hidden threads, they are invisible to our eyes, to our understanding—until, perhaps a photograph, a whispered conversation late at night, a tear welling up and dropping from a memory—and then we catch a glimpse of the truth that we are made not only of the joys and choices and struggles that press in upon our daily consciousness but also of forgotten sorrows.

So it is with Charity Ann, the little girl who waited so long to come into our lives and then who departed, leaving behind only a few breaths of hopeful life before ascending to her eternal home. We named her as we saw her—Charity for Love and Ann for Grace. She was born at the sixth month of pregnancy during the bloody hemorrhage of a placenta previa. Today she would have survived—but not then. I have always felt that somehow this tiny life left us because she knew we needed her prayers and that she has been faithfully at her heavenly task for the decades when we needed her the most.

Charity Ann's departure ended forever my invincible self image. Wonder Woman was dead. I buried her with my child.

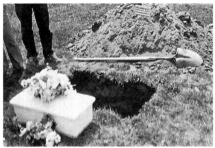

Charity Ann's grave.

The Fear Came upon Me

On November 11, 1981, I was sitting in my living room praying after a hard year. Charity Ann had died in the summer, and then there was the grief and a long recovery. She was my fourth child and my third C-section in five years. She lived just long enough to be issued a birth certificate and then, shortly after, a death certificate. While I stayed at home recuperating, Don and Sean carried her tiny body back to Indiana where all of our families assembled for a service of singing, scripture and prayer. They buried her at the foot of my mother's burial plot, and angels bore her away.

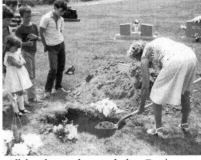

All family members, including Don's mom, Virginia York, take their turns in sending Charity home. That's the way we do it.

My body was worn out from all the surgeries and my spirit was whipped and beaten. This time I did not recover so quickly. I was not insightful about my body and did not know that all of the antibiotics from the surgeries had depleted vital nutrients from my body and weakened my immune system. I was just trying to get back on my feet and move on with my life.

While I sat there praying on that November day, I felt that God spoke to me quite clearly. I was frequently not sure whether I was hearing God or whether it was my own voice or my own ideas and desires that were coming to mind, but this time it wasn't something I would normally be saying to myself. The message was, "I'm moving your family. You will climb high mountains, walk through dark valleys, and swim deep rivers, but I will be with you." Quite frankly, I felt I had just been through a pretty dark valley, and at that time I couldn't imagine anything worse. Years later I would look back at this moment and know that it was a profound internal insight about what would happen to me and an assurance of grace. But at that time I could only wonder about it and record it in my Bible.

In February of 1982, within three months of this experience, Don received an invitation to apply for a position at the University of Chicago. We decided he should accept. In June we flew to Chicago to make final arrangements with the University and to scout housing and school possibilities for the kids. At that time we had the option of living either in Chicago near the Hyde Park campus or in Williams Bay, Wisconsin, near Yerkes Observatory. We had spent three years at Yerkes while Don was in graduate school, and we knew and loved the area. We had especially fond memories of beautiful Lake Geneva and the good times we shared with friends and faculty, some of whom were still at the observatory. I was looking forward to the new adventure and to visiting some favorite haunts by the lake.

On the day we were to visit Yerkes, I woke up in the morning with both legs partially numb to about the knees. I said to Don, "I don't know what's going on here. My legs feel so funny. It feels like I slept on them wrong and cut off the circulation or something." I stomped around the hotel room trying to restore circulation and dissipate the feeling of pins and needles prickling up and down my legs. Suddenly I felt like I was hit by a bolt of lightning. An enormous electric shock blasted through my body, throwing me on the bed and leaving me weak and shaking. I lay there dumbfounded for a moment while Don looked at me in astonishment. "I don't know what that was," I said shakily, trying to recover myself. "It felt like an electric shock. Are there any loose electrical cords in here?" Don did a quick check around the room and saw I was nowhere near an electric appliance or outlet. I lay there a moment and then sat up, rubbing my legs and frowning. Don sat beside me and put his arm around me, gently kissing my forehead. Then, to lighten the moment, he gave a little chuckle and said, "Well, lover, you'll just have to lay off of those alcoholic drinks before breakfast." "Hmm," I said. Totally puzzled, we struck out on a busy day of house hunting and appointments with faculty.

I was going downstairs into a basement rec room with a real estate agent when another blast went through my body. I missed my footing, grabbed the handrail, and slid down a couple of steps. Later, just at the moment when Don was introducing me to Lew Hobbs, one of the professors at the observatory, another lightning bolt went off, leaving me disoriented and embarrassed. Deep down I knew something was dreadfully wrong, but I put out a great effort to make a good impression on all Don's future colleagues.

The next day David Schramm, a famous astrophysicist and chairman of the Astronomy Department, showed us around the campus in Chicago. I felt like I was walking on numb stubs instead of legs, strangely disconnected from the earth. Ripples of sensation flowed upward with each step. I felt fatigued after a simple walk across the quads.

When we returned to Princeton, I went to bed hoping some rest would refresh me. The next morning when I stepped out the back door of our Tudor house, another blast went off and I fell down the stairs. We arranged for a baby sitter and went to see a neurologist, Dr. Enright, who immediately put me in the hospital.

Dr. Enright was reputed to be a good neurologist, but his bedside manner left something to be desired. The deciding factor for the hospital, as he phrased it, was, "When you can't feel yourself poop, there's probably something going on." They did a spinal tap, a procedure that gave me a million dollar headache and made me vomit my socks. I was checked into a room in the hospital across the hall from an old man who shouted four-letter words all night, increasing my impression that I had just landed in hell. In two more days I was numb to the neck. It felt like death was a giant anaconda, swallowing me feet first and digesting me a little at a time as I was sucked in by peristaltic waves. Soon my head would go down and everything would be black. The numbness was punctuated by jolting electric shocks. My nervous system was blowing up.

Wild sensations assailed my helpless body as I lay in my bed. Sometimes it was the anaconda, squeezing, loosening, tightening, engulfing. Sometimes I felt like I was encased in wet cement that was drying, cracking, splitting my skin, weighing my body down. I could tell my arms and legs to move if I concentrated very hard, but the result was unpredictable; they might or might not do what I told them. Soon I was unable to feed myself. The food was there on the tray, and my brain was telling my hands to pick it up, but my hands just lay there inert. The first time someone had to spoon feed me, I felt I was regressing back into childhood. Time was reversing and my body was failing me. What would happen next?

Each day six neurologists stood around my bed. One poked me with pins up and down my arms and legs. Another one ran a pointed stick up my feet from heels to toes. Another pinged an instrument like an oversized tuning fork and placed it on my body at various points to see if I could detect the vibrations. They also did other invasive, painful tests that failed to reveal any answers. At that time there were no MRI's to scan the brain for abnormalities indicating various neurological disorders; my body was a black box into which no one could peer. Lacking modern internal scanning devices, the six neurologists reminded me of the six blind men who tried to describe an elephant, each one seeing a different attribute and offering a different diagnosis. They were the experts of that day, but they were stumped. I was a mystery to the medical establishment.

It became obvious that I would not be going home any time soon. Don packed up our three youngest children, ages 5, 4, and 3, and sent them to Indiana to my parents' house for an indefinite stay. Our oldest son Sean stayed in Princeton with Don. I was an object of consternation and pity and prayer for hundreds of people. Friends came to see me and read scripture and prayed with me, but it was hard for them. No matter

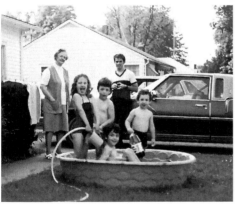

We sent our boys to stay with Grandma and Grandpa Hinds while I was in the hospital.

how much I tried to cheer them up, they usually left looking grim. One day my neurologist came in to see me, obviously stressed and nervous, smoking a cigarette. These were the days before smoking was banned from health facilities. I always thought Dr. Enright was a pretty hard-as-nails type guy, sometimes swearing while he was poking me with pins. Pinprick—"Damn." Pinprick—"Shit!" He stubbed the cigarette out in the ashtray on the bed stand and happened to look up on my bulletin board to see the pictures of our smiling, happy kids. He stopped, leaned against the stand for a moment, staring at the pictures, and then he looked at me with his mouth pursed and his forehead wrinkled in consternation. Tears came to his eyes. He blurted out, "I'm so sorry!" and fled the room.

Things were not looking good. It wasn't just Dr. Enright, it was everyone who came to see me. I could see it in their worried frowns, their inability to look me in the eye; I could hear it in their overly optimistic encouragements and in the catch in their voices when they prayed with me. I didn't have much else to do but read the signs, and the signs were all bad.

Even so, there was something inside of me that rose up to reject the worst possibilities and to defy a destiny that was too horrible to contemplate. I believed, in spite of it all, that I would be all right. I began to draw on all the faith I ever had, faith in the love of God and Christ, faith in resurrection, faith in the Spirit, faith that I had lived a good life and would surely reap the reward of a faithful, righteous servant of God, faith that God would not abandon me. I believed I had a God who is able to make me all right, and I believed wholeheartedly that God would. Everyone was fasting and praying for me. I had prayed so many people out of desperate situations that I felt sure God would get me out of this one. Faith may be tested, but "Keep the faith, God will bring you through!" That's what I believed, even in spite of knowing that God does not always do things in exactly the way we expect. I believed that God was my ticket out. I just didn't know I had a ticket for a very long ride, and I didn't know where I was going.

Do-Be-Do-Be-Do

I recall having a good laugh when I heard the joke about the three philosophers arguing the meaning of existence. The first asserted that he believed Socrates was right when he claimed that "to do is to be." The second sided with Plato in arguing that "to be is to do." The third replied that he held with Frank Sinatra on this point: "Do-be-do-be-do."

I was faced with the meaning of existence as I lay in my hospital bed and was surprised that I had not confronted it before in terms of the being-doing dilemma. For me, having grown up as a Christian in a Christian family, faith was always demonstrated by doing. To be a Christian is to do. From my earliest remembrance I was a Miss and then a Mrs. with a mission. Sometimes I struggled with precisely what I should do at a particular time, but never with the fact that I must do something for God. Suddenly, however, I was unable to do any work at all, for myself or others. Although I did believe God would get me out of this trouble, I didn't know how God was going to do it, and I couldn't predict when it was going to happen. Ghosts of possibilities chased each other through my mind, some spooking me, some horrifying me. I heard about a woman my age who, more than a year before, had mysteriously gone into the same condition as I, only a little worse, and she was still that way—a terrifying prospect.

What had seemed an adventure of moving to a new life in Chicago suddenly became a nightmare. The questions engulfed my mind like the paralysis that engulfed my body: What would I *do* in Chicago? What would I *do* with my children? What would I *do* about my shopping, my housework, errands for the children, about the long business trips my husband frequently took to the far corners of the world? What would I ever be able to *do* for God? The possibility fleetingly occurred to me that I might not ever be able to *do* anything again. If that happened, what would I *be*? I chased this ghost firmly from my mind.

In the meantime, after all three younger children went to live with Grandma and Grandpa in Indiana, I was moved from the hospital to a rehabilitation floor in Merwick. I considered Merwick, a nursing home in the middle of Princeton, to be the place where they put you before you die. For many people it was true. Black body bags going out the front door, followed by pale, weeping relatives, were not an uncommon sight. I was being sent there for an "undetermined" time.

My check-in day was one of the grimmest days of my life. The ambulance ride from the hospital was torturous, with each bump sending shocks through my body. At Merwick they put me in a wheelchair and wheeled me up to a small, empty cafeteria to wait for my room. I was unable to sit upright, so I slumped over the table with my head in my arms, exhausted from the ride. After a few moments I slowly rolled my head to the side and opened my eyes half way. There was a homemade tagboard sign on the wall with little magazine pictures pasted on it around a message that I'm sure was supposed to be encouraging to the residents: "Everyone has handicaps. On some people they show." I thought of my poor, inert, painful body and knew that my handicaps were all hanging out there for anyone who would cast an eye in my direction. I wept, silently, mournfully. Would I always be this way? I wiped my tears on my hospital gown, closed my eyes and fell asleep with my head on the cold, hard table.

Later, after check-in, I took up residence in a double room with Catherine, a woman whose body had been horribly injured in a severe automobile accident. She had been in therapy at Merwick for six months. She was a dear woman, and I was happy for her good company. I could have done much worse. The old lady across the hall swore at people all day long, especially at the nurse who had a habit of asking her daily in a sickening, motherly tone, "Can I wash your little girl parts now?" I figured the nurse deserved some swear words for treating a grown woman like a child and plotted how I would bust her in the jaw if she dared question me in such a fashion. My little girl parts were all grown up, thank you! Others on the floor were recovering from strokes, neurological diseases or severe accidents.

Life assumed a bizarre regularity, consumed by personal hygiene, friends and family coming in to visit and feed me, and physical and occupational therapy. Taking a bath required so much energy that I needed a long rest afterwards. Therapy confronted me with an endless variety of tasks I could not perform. I remember the day I tried to write my name and the scrawl went all over the page. Walking between two bars took all the strength I could muster, and then I would collapse. Nights, which should have been a refuge for refreshment, were punctuated by relentless medical routines. All night long nurses in combat boots patrolled the halls, shining floodlights in everyone's eyes, determined that no one would get a good night's sleep while they were on guard.

During the long periods of rest between the activities of daily living, I had plenty of time to lie in bed and think. I pondered what I needed to do to be healed. My Christian experience had taught me that God's ability to work is often limited by a person's ability to let go of old thoughts and patterns and be open to new possibilities. I thought back to the message God gave me that we were going to move and that I would climb high mountains, walk through deep valleys and swim deep rivers. What I was experiencing now was more than I bargained for. I knew I was unwilling to go to Chicago, and I knew that the reason was fear. I did not know what would happen to me and what I would do there. How would I take care of my family? But the time was critical for us to let Chicago know whether we were coming or not.

One Saturday night, after I had been at Merwick for about three weeks, I had a phone conversation with a trusted friend who reframed the question. After a long conversation, she said, "Anna, what does God want you to do?" I remembered the words I had heard, "I'm moving your family. I will be with you." I felt in my heart that God wanted us to make the move. I gripped the phone, took a deep breath and said, "God wants me to go to Chicago." That night I decided I would take a leap of faith and go to Chicago even if I went as a stewed vegetable.

The following day, Sunday, I began to feel peculiar power surges in my body—not the cruel lightning blasts—but good, healthy feelings of strength. The circuit breakers in my body began to turn back on. First I took steps in the hall without falling down. That was a major achievement! Then I picked up my utensils and awkwardly began to feed myself. On Monday doctors began showing up again in my room, and by Tuesday I was cruising up and down the hall with no walker or cane. On the third day I took a victory walk—down the hall, out of the building and around the garden. My stunned physiatrist watched me walk and proclaimed it was a miracle. She called in my neurologist, who poked me with more pins, of course, and pronounced me ready to go home. In a state of considerable astonishment, I went.

I honestly don't know what happened at that time that caused my body to rejuvenate, and I don't think anyone else could answer that question either. I would later discover that MS is extremely capricious and can relapse and remit in a great variety of bizarre patterns. Perhaps that's what it was—just a spike amidst a lot of undecipherable noise in the data of my disease. On the other hand, perhaps it was, as I believed at the time, God's miraculous response to my step of faith and obedience. Recent research indicates that feelings of hope can set off a cascade of healing hormones in the body. Perhaps that's what it was. Whatever it was, a new phase of my life had begun. We would move to Chicago within the month. Questions of how to do everything that needed to be done for this new development were so overwhelming that the deeper questions of how to do for God and be for God and for all the people in my life could only be strangers, vaguely flitting past the windows of my mind. I banished them from my presence. When physical strength comes in, spiritual insight often flees.

Will Power Is Not Enough

I walked out of the hospital, but I couldn't walk far. My body was like one of the kids' battery-operated robots when the battery was running low. The arms and legs are ready to go, but there just isn't enough energy to make them move except in slow, jerky, unpredictable ways. My healing and the initial thrill of leaving the hospital gave me enough energy to get me moving, but my strength fell far short of what I needed to accomplish the enormous task ahead of us.

Our house had three stories and a basement, four kids, three roomers and mountains of stuff that had to be sorted and moved. I would have been a good candidate for one of those massive modern makeovers they demonstrate on TV these days, the ones where they throw all of your stuff on the lawn and insist you get rid of fifty percent. My mountain of junk had to be climbed, and I had to do it as a cripple. Devastating electric shocks surged through me whenever I so much as ran my hand across a sheet. The hot July weather made me numb and tingly from head to foot, and even small activities brought on paralyzing exhaustion. No one could explain this to me because I never had a diagnosis. Fortunately, the children were still with Grandpa and Grandma. An army of friends helped with packing, throwing out trash, and organizing a yard sale. Finally, I left the worst of it for Don, and Sean and I flew to Indiana to join the rest of the family. It was late summer of 1982.

We migrated to Chicago before it evolved into the beautiful, garden-filled city it is today. Chicago was foreign territory for a country girl like me. The Hyde Park community, located fifty blocks south of the Loop on Lake Michigan, encompasses approximately one square mile and has a population of about 50,000 people with highly diverse ethnic backgrounds. The southeast corner of the neighborhood is anchored by the famous Museum of Science and Industry. Within Hyde Park's borders are the University of Chicago, its complex of hospitals, and several seminaries of various kinds, all of which draw students and teachers from around the world. The north, south and western sides of the neighborhood at that time touched on poverty- blighted and crime-ridden areas into which few Hyde Parkers dared to set foot.

I was awed by the city, its huge buildings, the noisy traffic, and the crowds of people thronging the streets. For this reason, I was relieved that the Chairman of the Astronomy Department offered to let us rent his house for a greatly reduced rate. The house was located on three spacious lots in Kenwood, a quiet and beautiful neighborhood on the north edge of Hyde Park. I thought living in this big house would ease the transition to the city for us. It saved me from the horrible fear I had of living in a small apartment in a high rise where the children would not be able to run out the door to play. Furthermore, I knew it was big and spacious enough to begin a ministry to university students similar to the one we had in Princeton. I was already planning what I would do with my life and for God.

The big, colonial-style house was incredible in every way. It was built around 1911, when Hyde Park was a luxurious suburb for the rich and famous. It boasted its own coach house, servants' quarters, and three and a half floors of living space. The basement was equipped with an enormous playroom, a wine cellar, and a fire-belching furnace that tended to go on the blink in sub-zero weather. The furnace was only one of many things that needed repair in this monster domicile.

Shortly after we moved in, we discovered there were already several other permanent residents. I learned that some of them, mice in numbers worthy of the Pied Piper and cockroaches the size of a VW bus, just came with the city territory. The exterminator and I came to be on all too familiar terms as we fought back the jungle to make a healthy space for ourselves. As the extermination program took hold, smells of death and decay began to emanate from the walls, and one day a baby mouse careened drunkenly across the atrium floor in front of my eyes to find refuge under the throw rug. Too much!

The inner invasion was bad enough, but one morning I was shocked to go outside and see big orange signs posted to our trees with pictures of voracious-looking rats on them. Our neighborhood was quarantined for pets because Mayor Jane Byrne's "rat patrol" was putting poison out to kill the beasts! Chicago's mutant denizens of the sewers were hot topics of conversation among neighbors and even at some Hyde Park dinner parties. I discovered I had the same exterminator as Mohammed Ali, who lived in an imposing mansion a block away. It was my exterminator who told me a perhaps apocryphal story about Ali's pink plush bedroom with a picture of the champion in boxing regalia hanging above the bed.

We also had squirrels in our attic—a whole army of them. When we moved in, we stored most of our boxes in the attic, and the squirrels proceeded to turn them into their own personal condominium, hiding their nuts and acorns in my pots and pans and building nests in the packing paper. Every attempt to evict these little rascals or plug the attic holes failed, and they even took to scolding us in chorus every time we popped our heads in the attic door. The exterminator wanted thirty dollars per squirrel to trap and export them, with no guarantee that ten others wouldn't take their places the next day. Finally, at a prayer meeting, someone undoubtedly under divine inspiration suggested the harmless and effective remedy of mothballs. Squirrels don't like the smell. We used them, and the squirrels left overnight.

But the biggest non-paying guest of all was Chuck, the owner's Great Pyrenees dog, which we had agreed to keep for him while he made permanent arrangements about his house. Chuck's natural, boisterous energy was untamed by any formal training, a situation that "unleashed" him to create constant canine chaos. The back gate couldn't hold him, and we often had to wrestle him back from his neighborhood romps, during which he terrified innocent old ladies and ate Volkswagen beetles. Chuck also dug giant excavations that exposed the foundations of the house in the back yard. After a rain they would turn into big muddy swimming pools for dog and children alike. Indoors, there was so much of Chuck's dog hair in every corner that I started collecting bagsful of it to spin into yarn. I figured in a year I'd probably have enough to make a matching hat, coat and mittens. Our adventures with Chuck could provide folly enough for our own comic strip.

Unfortunately, I had gone from Wonder Woman to Wimpy Woman. We were facing the biggest task of our lives, establishing a new life for a whole family, and my body had decided to go on vacation. Lightning bolts periodically exploded inside me, leaving me weak and shaking. Before my illness, no job had been too big, no challenge too great. Now, getting breakfast was an Olympic trial. Doing dishes was facing the firing squad. Every task I did took a long time and required rest periods and great perseverance. For seven months after my initial attack I was unable to drive except for occasional short distances. Chicago's infamous potholes, known to swallow whole trucks in a single gulp, didn't help any. They made a trip in the car into an experience rather like riding the Shockwave at the Six Flags amusement park.

We tried valiantly to make life "normal" for the children, getting them into activities and playgroups and helping them keep up with schoolwork. At the same time, I was hardly able to even hug the children without setting off electric shocks in my body. Tasks were lined up on a mile-long NOW! priority list. Don, who had always pitched in with all housework and childcare tasks, was overwhelmed by a new job and by the need to do, in addition, all the jobs I had always done. At a time when I most needed to *do,* I was the least able to do anything at all.

At the same time, I continued to attempt things that normal people would have found challenging. I developed a student ministry through a group on campus, opening our home for hospitality and special events. I couldn't get it into my head that I needed a different lifestyle. For me weakness was something to be overpowered—or denied. Faith would be affirmed by physical prowess. God didn't want me to be this way. Since my physical problems had not been identified, I had no idea how to live with them and manage them. My nature, geared to perseverance, was completely unsuited to patience. I repeatedly drove myself to the edge of endurance, thinking that by so doing I would gain strength and stamina. I asserted my faith over every obstacle. Adrenalin carried me over the Everest of the moment, and fatigue flung me over the precipice on the other side. My expeditions into frustration always left the home camp in disarray. The more I tried to be an overcomer, the more soundly I was defeated and the longer it took me to recover and resume tasks I could handle in managing our lives. The higher I tried to climb, the deeper Don had to shovel to dig us out of the mess. I became an expert in cracking my head up against the wall of reality.

Finally, I cracked my head a little too hard when I took in a roomer. I was incorrigibly drawn to down and outers, and Karla's credentials on this score were impeccable. She was a student at the University and a certified paranoid schizophrenic who consumed huge amounts of my time and energy. She lived with us for several months until she was back on track academically and had learned how to balance a checkbook. Her room, which once looked like an explosion in a laundry factory, took on more the semblance of normal human habitation, and she was finally ready to move out into an apartment on her own. The rest of us were ready for a long vacation. My experience with Karla made me realize I was no longer physically able to handle the kind of work I had done before, helping people rehabilitate their broken lives. My own was broken enough.

After Karla moved out, I took a rest, and my health took a turn for the better. The sensations in my body calmed down and my strength improved. I began to lead a much more normal life than I had since the big attack. I began to think that I had put a horrible nightmare permanently behind me. I didn't know that one of the cruelest characteristics of my disease was that it could disappear and then suddenly leap out again like a dragon from the dark. My eternal optimism (or robust denial) caused me to enter the fray of life too fast and too hard. I never gave myself an opportunity to really recover before I launched out into a new enterprise.

As soon as I began to feel better, I looked around at my options. I was stuck with the idea that in order to be worthwhile life must be lived in the context of an overarching mission. I was fatally goal oriented. I had been deeply disappointed as a child that I could never be a preacher or missionary because the church I belonged to at the time disallowed such callings to females. In a way, I spent the first forty years of my life trying to discover what my mission was, considering the limitations of my feminine body. My mission had to be service to both God and people. Failure to accomplish tangible results was more than just not quite making it—it was failure as a Christian and, for me, failure as a human being.

I looked around for a new goal and saw that Don had taken an interest in researching the relationship between science and religion. He wanted to be able to share his insights through public lectures, and I picked up his mission as my own. My new energy vented itself in intellectual pursuits I would never have dreamed of before. I had always said I hated science and had felt I was bad at it. Now I plunged into history and philosophy of science and it became fascinating to me. I audited some philosophy classes at the University of Chicago and wrote papers on science and religion. The creationist conflict was bursting on the national media, and Don and I wanted to address the issues. I began regularly attending the classes and seminars of the Hyde Park science and religion group that met at the Lutheran School of Theology and that drew a distinguished clientele of professors and students from around the Chicago area. I was the least distinguished and learned; nevertheless, I found the group highly stimulating. After a couple of years, I even presented one of my own papers to the group.

I put my new learning to use by writing science and religion speeches that Don gave at colleges around the country through the Shapley lectures, sponsored by the American Astronomical Society. I began to think seriously about doing a master's degree and then perhaps a doctorate, focusing on science and religion issues. I was accepted and had my heart set on a program at the Lutheran School of

Theology for the fall of 1987. Even if my body would not support great physical exertion, I could employ my mind as the doer and achiever in my personality and perhaps fulfill the elusive mission I believed God had for me. I launched myself into *yet another* life mission.

If I had looked back, I might have seen that my life missions were beginning to accumulate something like the nine lives of a cat. First was teaching, three years; then social work in a home for delinquent boys, six months; then reading and writing in feminist theology, two years; then Bible teaching, two years; student ministry, four years; and now science and religion. How long would that last? Being a wife and mother was a serious occupation for me and one I pursued with enthusiasm and reverence; however, it did not seem to satisfy my desire to reach out and touch my world.

Before long other circumstances in our lives began to intrude. We had moved into a big condo on a lease-purchase arrangement and, as the deadline for purchase was looming, we needed money to close the deal. I went to work on a temporary basis, doing office work in the University hospitals. The shock of Mom working was not easy for my family. I was supposed to be there for everything, carrying forgotten lunches to school, running errands, picking up all the loose ends. When Don's grant proposals were due, I often typed them on crash deadlines. I tried to continue doing all this and a job too, and my health began to crack. My nervous system started short-circuiting again, and I developed a limp. My stamina and energy declined seriously, and I had to cut back to working part time. I could barely drag myself to the office for a half day and drag myself back home again. Small tasks once again became huge chores. My healing was seeping away like water through sand.

I am astonished at the potency of human will. It is like an engine that is able to move a much larger, inert vehicle—as long as it has enough fuel. In this case the fuel was my sense of personal identity, which was largely defined in terms of being able to do and achieve. I had driven my car far and hard, but by the fall of 1987, my health was still declining, and my engine of will power was barely running. Negotiations on our apartment should have gone quickly, but they dragged out for more than a year. Worry weighted my spirits down, and I finally realized that it would be impossible for us to carry the financial burden of my going to school as long as the problem went unsettled. I cancelled my school plans, and my dreams of doing a doctorate died, never to revive again. Immediately, I plunged into depression.

It seemed like events were manipulating me and that I couldn't control anything in my life, no matter how much I wanted to and no matter how hard I tried. I decided to give in and see a neurologist for the first time in five years. My experience in Princeton had been so horrible that I had avoided doctors like the plague. After a round of state-of-the-art tests, some of which had been unavailable five years earlier, Barry Arnason, a renowned neurologist at the University of Chicago, told us I had multiple sclerosis.

Future Shock

Multiple sclerosis. You might think I would take the news fairly calmly. After all, I had already lived with the disease for at least five years. No, there had been no name attached to it. I could always fool myself into believing it would go away tomorrow. Now the monster within had a fearful name, and the ugly beast roiled inside me, stirring raw depths, threatening to give birth to a life form I hated, dreaded, and pitied.

First I thought of my future. All I could see was wheelchairs, crutches, and a deformed, struggling body, the worst expressions I had seen or knew about the disease. I remembered my experience with MS patients a few years earlier at the hospital outside Washington, D.C. I recalled how I had said to God, "Of all the things that could happen to me, please, Lord, don't let it be this!" When I heard the words "multiple sclerosis" applied to myself, I felt my worst nightmare had come true.

I tried to confront my fears by arming myself with the latest information about the disease. I went to the bookstore and bought a book about multiple sclerosis. Reading about MS initially encouraged me to some extent. There are about 350,000 people in the United States with MS, about one in a thousand of the whole population. Although it is a horrible, crippling disease for many people, others pursue fairly normal lifestyles. About thirty percent have no visible expressions of the disease, and many don't even know they have it. About forty percent must use some kind of physical aids such as crutches, canes or other devices. The final thirty percent are restricted to home or institution. Grasping at straws, I mentally slotted myself into the first category, those with no *visible* symptoms, refusing to accept the possibility of the other two. I remembered the sign that said, "Everyone has handicaps. On some people they show." I didn't want mine to show! Unfortunately, it was not long before I was in the last category, those who are confined at home.

MS is insidious, capricious, and completely unique to each individual. It may affect any part of the nervous system and, therefore, any part of the body and its functions. Unpredictability is one of its most frustrating characteristics. The cause is unknown, but it is suspected that most people acquire it before age twenty, even though it may not show up until much later in life. Infections and stress often accompany onset of episodes.

MS can be either progressively degenerative or can be expressed in a relapsing-remitting pattern. I had the relapsing-remitting type, which means that one has "exacerbations" during which the disease and its symptoms get worse. These are followed by periods of remission during which one can either recover completely or possibly be left with residual symptoms. Although it is common for exacerbations to begin and remit within a month, they might last much longer. Some people may have only one or two exacerbations in their entire lives. Some may have repeated small ones. Others may have several, large, debilitating exacerbations. There is no way of predicting the course of any individual's disease. Some have no pain at all. Others, like me, may have excruciating pain. Partial or complete blindness, incontinence, shaking, weakness, crippled limbs, chronic fatigue, numbness, and extreme sensitivity to heat and cold are all possible manifestations of the disease. Symptoms in any individual may be quite different from one episode to another, and sudden, dramatic remissions sometimes occur. There is no known cure, although there are now drugs that significantly change the course of MS. These drugs were not available, however, until about 1994, twelve years after my massive attack in 1982.

As I learned more about the disease, and as I became weaker, I experienced "future shock," thinking of all the possibilities of living as a crippled person. My mind was filled with questions and fears. At first these questions were all encapsulated in one big, unfocused question: "What will I do? O, dear God, what will I do?" Then, with some time and reflection, the questions sorted themselves out into individual little power packs, each delivering its own special, cruel punch. Will my looks be marred? How can I hide my problems? Will my family still love me? Will my spouse be true and faithful and helpful? Will my children be embarrassed and despise me? Will I lose my job? Will my friends still come around and call me? How bad will this thing get? Will it cause me to die early? Will I even want to live?

I realized how precious my future is to me, how important it is to my feelings of self worth. I began to understand that when I think of what I will do tomorrow, or next week or next month or two years from now, I engage in a process of self-perception and self-definition. I help myself decide what my capacities and goals are for the future. I dream, and, because I dream, I have a vision of the future that I may be able to actualize. I envision possibilities, and when I envision them, I prepare myself to reach for them. I search inside myself for my potentials, with the hope of realizing them. I engage in a process of defining who and what I am as a human being. When I think of the future, I am also meditating on God's possibilities for me and for what I will do in my life for God. In this sense, pondering my future doings helps me define my place in the world and my reason for being here.

With the diagnosis of MS, I saw my future reeling wildly, like a satellite out of control. I peered out small windows on a macabre universe. Strange faces and shapes leered and beckoned at me, silently hooting and jeering, then passing in the dark. It occurred to me that if I had MS, I could make no long-range plans. The disease could change them without my consent any time it chose. I was the raw material of caprice. I was losing my future. As I advanced, my future receded. As I hoped, it shriveled. As I planned, it crumbled. If I had prayed and believed and had hope and faith and apparent healing in my previous illness, and I still had the monster within, what could I do now that would save me? I went into mourning for my future.

Worst of all, mission control seemed to have abandoned my project like a satellite with a failed mission. I was launched, tracked for a while, then aborted. Words began forming and articulating themselves deep in my spirit, words I had rebuked as faithless in other troubled souls, words that carried guilt, defeat, and shame, words directed at a God I thought I knew but didn't at all: "Damn it all to hell! This shouldn't happen to me! I'm too good! I played the game, and I don't deserve this! Who do you think you are, God!?"

Demolition of the Past

"What's done is done." That's an old saying that on the surface would seem to be true. How can anyone go back in time and change what has already happened? Time seems to have an arrow, pointing always into the future. We live by the arrow of time and depend on it; our whole lives are structured by it. We are born, we live, we die, all according to a normal progression of time. Our watches and clocks keep us moving forward in time, making appointments, meeting deadlines, working toward expectations.

Increasing disability and the diagnosis of multiple sclerosis revealed to me the falsity of the maxim, "What's done is done." What's done is not really done at all, not in our minds. History scholars know this is true. People recreate history all the time to suit their own designs. They do this by hiding what is embarrassing or doesn't suit their purposes; by embellishing marginal events that enhance a point of view; by erasing whole periods of history through book burning or destruction of documents; by ignoring the obvious; or by reinterpreting past events in light of new developments. I was surprised to find that I do this on a personal level all the time and that I have indeed done it my whole life. It took me forty-two years to construct my history; it took only a few months to demolish it, and along with it much of what I recognized as myself.

I had always perceived myself as a basically healthy person, even, as I mentioned before, somewhat of a Wonder Woman. Life was always exciting, full of challenge, and, perhaps best of all, full of mission. I lived to do things for others. Health was a gift of God, and if I became ill, God's healing was also a gift. With increasing weakness and disability, I began to look back and question all of my previous self-perceptions. Had I really been a healthy person? The book I had read about MS said that most people get the disease before they are twenty. I looked back to see if there was any evidence earlier in my life of the coming tragedy. Yes, there was the episode on the drama trip in my sophomore year of college. My nervous system had blown up then with spectacular fireworks. I had spent some days in the hospital and had dropped out of school for a semester. The freaky Kansas incident, undiagnosed at the time, was chalked up to stress. Then there were the strange sensations I had in my third year of teaching high school. That had been called stress also. The signs were there. I hadn't read them, and neither had anyone else. My illness was woven into the fabric of my whole life. I had drastically misjudged myself. I had interpreted my own history to please myself, disregarding vital evidence and burning the documents that didn't agree with my own point of view.

Other musings confirmed my mistaken self-image. I had spent three years researching and writing a manuscript on male and female as God's image. I had come to a personal belief that females as God's creation are intended to be strong, equal companions with males. I had thought that through prayer, faith, the love of my husband, and Christ's gift of redemption females could become what God intended us to be. I thought I could be such a woman. After years of faithfulness, devotion, and hard work, I looked at the physical wreck of myself and realized I must have made a terrible misjudgment. Perhaps it was true after all that women are the "weaker sex" and are intended to be dependent and submissive, weak at the core.

I looked at the social self that I had known in the past, a self that I had loved and enjoyed, and it was like looking at a photograph of a distant relative. I had heard from other handicapped people that friends instantly disappear when a handicap appears. I thought that was crazy. Certainly not *my* friends. But I was the one who was wrong. Prior to this new exacerbation in 1987, my neurological handicaps had been invisible, and I had little experience of being obviously handicapped. Now no one could miss seeing my handicaps, and they became social as well as physical. I would never have believed I could be so alone, I who had always been there for everyone else. Many people didn't know what the problem was. Others didn't know what to do, so they did nothing, not even call me. When I appeared at a church or social gathering, people would often avoid me or pass by without looking at me in order to avoid embarrassment. I was the one who had to flag people down and be joyful and strong and vivacious, for their sakes. It wore me out.

The more I thought about the past, the less I was able to make any connection at all between the person I was now and the person I had been before. I looked into the grave where I had buried Wonder Woman, along with my child Charity Ann, and I mourned her. I mourned her energy, her joy, her freedom, her independence. I mourned her capacity to love and give and share and explore. I mourned her creativity. I mourned her ability to throw parties and care for her family. I mourned her ability to go to the grocery store, clean house, wash dishes, and go to a third grade play. I mourned her ability to walk down steps and get in a car. I mourned her ability to go anonymously through a crowd without seeing averted glances of pity.

Yes, Wonder Woman was dead. The past was dead. When you don't know who you have been, how can you have any idea of who you are now?

Denial of the Present

The present moment can be the cruelest of all times for a disabled person. *Now* is a perpetually crying child, clamoring with its needs, asserting its truth, demanding attention. As disability increased, I pursued numerous strategies in dealing with this fretful child. Most of them failed. They failed because I hated her, ignored her, or denied her existence. Only when I embraced Now and called her my own did she respond with quietness and love. But we wrestled with each other for a long time before we developed a working relationship.

Dealing with this present moment was the last thing I wanted to do. I denied that I was getting physically worse. Even when I could no longer get to the bathroom or kitchen, I refused to admit what was happening to me. My feet burned fiercely as though they were being roasted over hot coals. The slightest touch on the soles was excruciatingly painful. As a consequence, I could only walk a few steps at a time. Sometimes I crawled; sometimes I just didn't go anywhere at all. I had to lie on the bed with the bottom of my feet sideways or up to avoid pain. I couldn't go outside, because I couldn't get to the car without being carried. Still, I stubbornly clung to my delusions. I thought as long as I wasn't in a wheelchair I was okay.

For me, as with many disabled people, dealing with the problems of living each moment can be an overwhelming task. Doing everything is hard. Just think about cutting a finger or spraining a wrist or ankle and the many kinds of adjustments one must make for even small injuries. One must learn to do things in different ways, relearning simple activities, adjusting habits of eating, drinking, dressing and bathing. But my disability was much worse. Sometimes it was a matter of whether I would be able to do anything at all, even the most basic functions of life.

I discovered that what I missed most was the exercise of spontaneous choice. I couldn't suddenly decide to have a cup of tea or a snack—I couldn't reach the stovetop or the cookies. I couldn't decide to run out to the store for a gallon of milk or to go to a PTA meeting. I couldn't run upstairs to print something off on my neighbor's laser printer. I had to wait, sometimes for things I really needed, until someone was there to help. I had to plan and arrange my schedule around others. Sometimes I would sit in my chair scheming about how I could do something I wanted to do on my own, even something small such as getting a box of clothes off of an upper shelf. Repeatedly, even simple tasks spoke to me in derogatory, whining tones: "You are *dependent.*"

Dependency evoked a range of feelings in me. Sometimes I felt inadequate, sometimes I felt frustrated, sometimes I felt downright inhuman. The present moment was no longer mine to enjoy, to mold, to create—or even to do what was necessary to survive. What I would do during a day might be unfamiliar, unattractive, unfulfilling, even disgusting. The normal routines and expectations of a day were shattered by pain or by impossible tasks. Choice was supplanted by necessity. Spontaneity was the victim of dependency. The challenge of living was elbowed aside by the demands of existing.

Although my pain, physically, psychologically and spiritually, was great, I had to admit I was more fortunate than some. I was not alone in my striving to cope with the present moment, nor was I alone in trying to mask its ugly face. I had my loving husband Don. Once again, the burden fell on him. Don and I both felt it was important to keep things as "normal" as possible for the children, thinking and hoping I might snap out of my problems any day. Everyone's schedules and activities were stubbornly maintained. Of course, I recognized the load Don was carrying and was greatly burdened as I saw him struggle. My response was to deny further my own needs, hoping to relieve at least part of the pressure on him. I kept retreating from the center of activity, partly because I couldn't handle the stress of being there and partly to diminish the problems I created when I was in the middle of the bustling family life. I didn't like intruding on activities with my needs. My office-sunroom became my world. I had recently begun doing marketing research for my neighbor upstairs, and I escaped into my work, appeasing myself by saying that at least I could earn some money while I was sitting around at home.

Some philosophers design grand sayings about the fleeting nature of time and the elusiveness of the present moment. Perhaps time flies in this way for some people, but I know from my own experience that when the past is odious and the future unthinkable, the present moment can be a vacuum, a void, a lacuna. It can suck you into nothingness and roll you like an empty, forsaken, far-flung planet. Escape is desirable—but to where? Into past comforts or future fantasies? Into anger and disillusionment, self-pity, self-centeredness, pills, alcohol?

I had barely begun examining my options for escape when I was suddenly confronted with a hard dose of reality. It was on a Good Friday that Don said to me, "Anna, today we're going to get you a wheelchair." For me a wheelchair was the symbol of ultimate loss of control and an acknowledgment of defeat. It seemed to me like it was a Good Friday with no Easter to come.

Alone and Lonely

Loneliness surprised me. Before I was ill, I really didn't know what loneliness was. I had children, babies, students, and counselees around me twenty-four hours a day. I was never alone, and I liked it that way. But increasing disability began to isolate me. Loneliness crept into that isolation, into that space in my life that was once occupied by friends and activities, and began to exercise its guerilla tactics on me. I came to realize that loneliness is an enemy with many faces. I became familiar with several of them.

One face of loneliness is isolation that comes through loss of community. This was probably the first form of loneliness I became aware of, and, because I have always been such a social creature, it was especially painful. I had always loved entertaining and making guests feel special by fixing elaborate Indian, Chinese, or other kinds of gourmet dinners. But as my disease progressed, I didn't have the stamina to fix the dinners, prepare the house or, sometimes, even to sit through an evening of challenging conversation. I missed such events, both for the interaction with other people and for the creativity and joy I always poured into them.

I also missed larger community involvement. I once was very active in the PTA and in the parents' organization for the swim team, and these activities gave me contact with a wide variety of interesting people and worthwhile projects. They not only satisfied a need for social interaction but also offered a channel for making a real contribution to the welfare of the community. But disability removed me from these activities. I found out that when you stop going out and doing things that most people are so busy with their own goings and doings that they don't have time to come in to see those who are shut in. After a while, relationships that are based on going and doing just tend to wither away.

The community that I missed most sorely was Christian community. After three or four years in Chicago, we began attending a small

Baptist church a few blocks away from our home. We liked the family closeness, the commitment to ministry with families, and the strong orientation toward social service. We especially liked that the church had a wide variety of people from various ethnic, national, and socioeconomic backgrounds. The pastor of the church was Susan Lockwood, one of the pioneers for women's ministry in the Southern Baptist Church. Susan's ministry was an inspiration to me. For a while I served on committees, aided in worship planning, and worked on projects of many kinds that gave me great joy. Unfortunately, I could no longer do this, nor could I always attend church. Extremely hot, cold, or bad weather often kept me in. Sometimes I just didn't have the energy to get there or the endurance to sit in the hard-backed seats. This meant, of course, that I was not only excluded from the fellowship of Christians, but also from the Lord's Supper. Our church was one that was strongly attuned to some issues of social justice, such as hunger and education for inner-city children, but they were not attuned to needs of the disabled and did not know how to minister to me. It was not yet the era of political correctness and outspoken demands for the rights of the disabled.

Once I was no longer able to do as much as I had done before in service and attendance, there was a weakening of relationships with those in the church. Even though we had a shared faith, it almost seemed like our deepest bonds were forged by our doings—whether it was for each other or the church or the community. But when my doing diminished, so did my bonds with others. I was not able to articulate this until several years later, but I began to experience in a poignant, personal way that *doing* is a poor foundation for building community. Was I no longer a valuable or even viable member of the community if I could not do as much as others or as much as I had done before? I didn't have any answers. I just had a great deal of pain from loneliness.

I also discovered that there is a loneliness that comes from having a different body than other "normal" people have. I experienced this body loneliness on at least two levels—a feeling of isolation from others and a feeling of strangeness about my own self. Body loneliness is quite a common affliction. Most of us experience it to some degree simply because we all have bodies that are unique and distinctive from one another. This kind of distinctiveness is especially important in relationships among different races because skin color is so obvious and supports so much stereotyping. Since I have lived in Chicago in a multi-ethnic community, my consciousness has been raised about such issues. As a disabled person, my body was different from other people's bodies, and I experienced the loneliness of being different. Visible handicaps set me apart, and I experienced from other people some of those expressions of rejection and alienation that are manifested in racial tension. Some of them were subtle and some were blatant. There were stares, averted glances, and looks of pity. I found myself reluctant to go to some places because I didn't want to experience the social stigma of being "deformed."

But more important was the feeling of loneliness that came from an almost universal lack of recognition and accommodation of my needs in a wide variety of settings. Lack of access made me feel really lonely and isolated. Handicap access to many places is not available even now, and when it is available, it is often not adequate. In 1987 it was much worse. Handicap access to some places might require a long wait to find someone with keys and information about how to get in. If it was cold outside, the wait could be painful. Access to a restaurant might be a half block away from the regular entrance, through long hallways, a kitchen, and up a grubby butler's elevator. Sometimes, even when the facilities were fairly accessible, it was still not a pleasant experience to use them. I recall going in a wheelchair to the Lyric Opera once with my friend Millie. The elevators to the balconies were crowded with pushy, fur-coated people, none of whom was willing to give me passage or space. They shouldered their way in front of me, and I had to wait for a later car.

But the worst access problem was handicapped parking. In my own community of Hyde Park I was finally unable to go anywhere because all the handicap parking spaces would be filled with healthy people who "just stopped for a minute" to take care of their business. When I confronted these people with my need, they usually became hostile and justified their behavior with their need for convenience. Loneliness came partly from my own feelings and inhibitions, partly from being blatantly shut out of places and activities other people take for granted, and partly from being pushed aside by stronger, thoughtless people.

My dysfunctional body also caused other kinds of loneliness. I was not always able to take care of my physical needs. Sometimes I couldn't get my food for myself because I couldn't reach the stove or the water faucet. Other times I couldn't reach items I needed to work with. I recall getting extremely frustrated when one of the children would carry my desk supplies away. Even if I knew where they had taken the pens or scissors or tape, it was impossible for me to get them because I couldn't get my wheelchair across a cluttered bedroom. When I was left alone and unable to meet my needs, I felt lonely and helpless indeed.

Another face of loneliness I saw was that of my own death. All humans must face the fear of death, and this often happens with the onset of severe physical problems or old age. As I saw it, mine would not be a sudden death, but a long, slow, painful death in which I would become more and more crippled with passing time until I finally became a human vegetable, cut off from all normal human communication and interaction. My prolonged illness and weakness and the prospect of a lonely death made me feel isolated in the face of an unthinkable future.

As I became familiar with the many faces of loneliness, I began to realize that loneliness had a number of macabre friends who wanted to spend time with me. One was self condemnation, my own sense of personal guilt about being disabled. Even though it was irrational,

I felt that perhaps I had done something to deserve my illness. Perhaps I had some serious personal defect that made me susceptible to this horrible disease. Such thoughts are common in general society, and those in churches are not immune to them. The sense of injustice when terrible things happen to people causes us to seek some behavioral or moral explanation, some hidden cause. Of course, when we look closely at ourselves and our past actions, we can always find some failings, even some garish flaws to assist our self accusation. But I couldn't pin down the root of my misfortune and didn't have the inner strength to dispel the condemning thoughts.

My feelings were exacerbated by the fact that I was no longer able to carry my accustomed share of responsibility for family care and sustenance. Quality of life for people around me deteriorated. This made me feel guilty—and even more so because I could not do anything about it. Guilt that I could not get rid of and could not share with anyone else was the arrow in the heart of my loneliness.

I was a cut-off portion of the body of humanity, not taking signals from the head, not functioning in tune with the rest of the body. My disease, my physical numbness, my neurological disintegration was a horrifying metaphor for my alienation from human community.

Does Anybody Know This Person?

Other people's opinion of me was an important part of the jigsaw puzzle making up my self-image. When the puzzle began breaking up, that part was lost among the pieces. What would people think of me? How could I interact with them? How could I put up a good front? How could I keep them liking me? This problem encompassed the closest members of my family and also every other relationship I had in the community.

As I look back, I see that this problem of what others might think of me was responsible for much of the huge effort I expended to keep going and doing all the things I had always done before. I'm not saying this was all bad. It was good in that it kept me persevering and interested in life. It was bad in that my fear of what other people would think disallowed an objective, constructive apprehension of my true situation. I kept hitting my head up against the wall of my physical limitations and falling back again, bruised and unable to accept a realistic life style.

This problem was never so acute as during one Christmas season when I was feeling very low. Christmas had always been a special time for me, and I tried to make it a special time for everyone else. I had always been right in the middle of all Christmas activities, making them happen, helping everyone have a good time, having a wonderful time myself. I loved shopping for exactly the right gifts and wrapping them to look pretty. I liked to have a family expedition to get the Christmas tree and then a special evening when the whole family and a few friends decorated the tree while sipping eggnog and sampling homemade candy and cookies. I loved arranging all the centerpieces exactly right and making sure all the boys' giant Christmas stockings were hung neatly across the fireplace. Each year we invited the campus chapter of Intervarsity over after Christmas caroling for hot chocolate, dessert, and an evening of fun and fellowship.

On this Christmas, however, I couldn't do any of that. I painfully missed my own involvement in everything. Even worse, however, was my horrible fear of what others would think of me, beginning with my children. Would they think I didn't even care? Not even enough to try? Would they think I was a morose and dull person because I couldn't join fully in the festivities? Would they want to go somewhere else to avoid being around me? How could I show them how much I cared?

Then there was the extended family. What if I sent money to the nephews and nieces instead of gifts? Would they think this was impersonal and that we didn't want to stay in touch with their needs and interests? As for my mother and father, sisters, and in-laws, we were unable to travel to see them at Christmas. Would they think we were just being stubborn and self-centered?

What about the campus Christian ministry? I had always enjoyed our projection of being a happy family with holiday traditions and homey joys. I thought we were being good family role models for them, as well as well as role models of Christian academicians. Now I couldn't have a party for them at all, or prepare a clever skit, or good food, or even go out on the steps to hear them sing. They all came in and stood around me. I didn't have any makeup on, and I was having a bad hair day. What would they think of me now? What would they think of our family? What would they think of my faith in God that I was stuck with a dreadful disease and not able to pray my way out?

I was also worried about what people would think about me at church. It was a small church. Would they think our family just didn't want to carry our share of the responsibilities there? Would they think I was no longer a worthwhile Christian?

One of the hardest problems for me was that I wanted to show Don how much I loved him and supported him in his work. Two or three times a year he had to prepare proposals for observing at various observatories or for grants from government agencies. The success of these proposals determined the success of his own research and his ability to financially support his students. It was one of the hardest things I have ever done to tell him I could no longer help him meet his deadlines. I feared that he would think I no longer loved him and cared about his work.

I also worried about what the people in Don's department would think. I wanted to be able to entertain them and respond to their hospitality to us. I wanted to be cordial to colleagues of Don's who were traveling through town, especially those who had entertained him on his many travels. Would they think we were ungrateful, unfriendly, uncaring? Would my failure affect Don's standing in the department?

Many of these questions were barely at the conscious level. At different times their ugly heads would pop up above the waves. I'd glance at them and push them back down again. Others of them swam before my eyes constantly, like ugly, primordial sea creatures waiting to take a bite out of me. They were symptoms of a personality in flux, in transition. I was no longer sure of who I was. At night I could hear a strange voice, asking me over and over again, "Who are you?" I could find no satisfactory answer. I just wanted to sit up and scream at the darkness, "Does anybody out there know this person?"

Victimized

One evening a few years ago I was returning home at about nine in the evening to our condo. I entered the first exterior door to the building and was about to enter the second when a man slipped in behind me and attacked me from the rear. He grabbed me with his arm around the neck, poked me in the ribs with something hard, and demanded my purse. Without thinking, I instantly began to scream bloody murder, my screams echoing in the small space between the doors. Fortunately, my screams frightened him, and he grabbed my purse and ran.

Being mugged between the doors of my own building gave me a terrible sense of being violated in a place I regard as sacred, my own home. Everyone in our building was upset and we analyzed why it happened—poor lighting outside, bushes someone could hide in, not being watchful enough. We took steps to prevent it in the future. We got a better alarm system, built a fence to secure the area next to the building, and put in motion-activated lighting.

In a similar way, my disease also attacked me from the rear in the sacred space of my body. It was strangling me and threatening my life. Unlike the measures we took to secure our building, I felt there was no way to guard against the MS monster lurking in the dark. Since I didn't know where it came from or how to guard myself against it, I could become a victim over and over again.

In fact, that's what happens with MS. Sometimes it's a bomb attack. You can be cruising along, going about your normal daily life, thinking everything is fine, and suddenly—BOOM!—it hits you like a lightning bolt, just as it had that time on the drama tour bus and at Yerkes Observatory. Other times it creeps up on you from the shadows, beats you up and takes your valuables. You don't know where it came from or what it will do to you. It happened over and over to me, sometimes a couple of times a year, but, as time went on, I would have up to six attacks a year. When it happened there was nothing I could do. I would go to the doctor, and he would prescribe steroids. A few times things got so bad I had to go to the hospital for intravenous injections. I became accustomed to having things "done" to my body—painful, invasive things. I accepted it because I didn't know what else to do. I took drugs every day, some of which alleviated symptoms and others that evened out my moods. It wasn't my fault. It's just the way it was.

Some friends gave me information early on about how diet might help me, but my doctor told me that there was nothing I could personally do through diet or exercise or any other way to prevent the disease or the attacks. Since my doctor was one of the leading researchers in the world on multiple sclerosis, I believed him and trusted him to handle my care. At the University of Chicago I was surrounded by people who were very much into the scientific paradigm. Making all decisions according to the latest research was the only rational way to do things. I did not explore other options because in the scientific paradigm in which we functioned it did not make sense. Furthermore, at that time, there was no Internet and information was not easily accessible.

I accepted the idea that disease "happens" to us from the outside and that we really can't do much for ourselves. Just as the problem comes from outside, the solution also comes from outside. Western medicine has the answers. It can solve all problems. We go to doctors and trust someone else to do all the thinking and strategizing for us. They give us magic pills that work on us in complicated ways we don't understand. They use huge, high tech machines to do tests we can't understand or interpret. We expect someone else to take responsibility for our problems and their treatment. If it's not successful or something goes wrong, we can blame someone else—and, even better, we can sue them and get someone else to pay for our pain!

Putting the responsibility somewhere else causes dependency. I was not aware that dependency causes a loss of personal will. Since it was not my fault or responsibility and I could do nothing about it, I stopped fighting. I just accepted my circumstances. I was developing a victim persona. The loss of will in the arena of personal health seeped out into the rest of my life like toxins through permeable cell walls. It became part of my muscles, my blood, my thoughts, my habits, my prayer life and my definition of relationship to God. Just as western medicine was working on me from the outside, God was also working on me from the outside. And, in the same way I didn't understand my disease, drugs, medicines and treatments, so also I didn't understand what God was doing. On the physical plane I submitted myself passively to the hands of doctors and western medicine. On the spiritual plane I submitted to an omnipotent God whose will was mysterious and inscrutable. I did not know at the time that, like all victims, my passive acceptance on the exterior was hiding anger that crouched like a feral lion deep inside. Years later, during the healing process, that the lion would come roaring out, showing its teeth.

Unknowing

We all want to make sense of what is happening to us, and we all want to relate to the world around us in ways that make us happy. Watching four children grow up, I was able to observe how each of them experimented with various behaviors and emotions to see how they could manipulate mom and dad, brothers, and other people to get the things they needed and wanted. Each child began to put together his own set of "rules" about what works best. One often stubbornly demanded his own way, and another occasionally took a good strong kick at a door. The youngest seemed to figure out from a very early age that the way to get what he wants is to be very agreeable, smile a lot, and do as much as possible for himself. As the children grew, they were assembling knowledge about themselves and their world that would undergird the rest of their life experience.

I also had developed a "rule book" or "book of knowledge" for my life. I developed it over many years from all my experiences as a person, and, throughout my daily life, I drew on it constantly to interpret my surroundings, decide on my responses, and design my plans. It was all built on the spirit of "rising" that was born into me, that had been modeled by my family and forbears and that had driven my life before my illness. But when MS took over, my book of knowledge became obsolete. Here are some of the rules I had relied on that no longer worked:

I can do it.
I can make myself do it.
God wants me to do it.
God will help me do it.
Working hard pays off.
There's an answer for everything.
God has the answer.
God wants me to know the answer.

I can figure it out.
I am supposed to be strong and healthy.
God wants me strong and healthy.
God has something for me to do.
God will make me strong so I can do it.

This set of rules didn't work because I no longer had the same body. Trying to use them was something like consulting a usage manual for a jet plane when you're driving a VW bus. I actually didn't know what kind of vehicle I was driving any more. My body had betrayed me. It had become a mystery to me. I recalled a VW bus we had owned several years previously. At some point the electrical system just went crazy. Sometimes the ignition wouldn't work at all, and other times the horn would blow when the ignition was turned on. Sometimes the windshield wipers would turn on at the same time as the lights. The best mechanics never did completely solve the problems, and we finally traded it in for a station wagon. Unfortunately, I couldn't trade in my body for a new model.

Not only did my own old rules not work, no one else had an instruction manual for my strange body or my new lifestyle. When I had studied science and religion, we often discussed on a theoretical basis the question of how much we can know through scientific investigation. Some people in our group seemed to believe science has or will have all the answers to everything. They feel the human body is a machine and that once we understand all the chemistry and physics we will be able to have complete control over it. Having a disease with no known cause and no known cure made me bump up against this issue as an acute, practical, everyday problem. I felt fortunate to have one of the world's experts as my doctor, but, even though there were some promising drugs, neither he nor any of his colleagues seemed to believe that an actual cure for MS would be forthcoming for many years. Confronting my own brokenness, I was skeptical and disillusioned that human knowledge would have any answers that would save me. It is a lonely feeling to live in a culture that thinks we have the answers to everything and to know from stark personal experience that we have answers to nothing at all.

Another kind of knowledge was failing me. Up to this time, I had always had pride in being a good self-analyst. I felt that the reason I was able to help other people was because I knew myself and could help myself. I had a good, solid upbringing by parents and family who loved me, with no unusual social, economic or personal traumas. I had a successful marriage and a beautiful family. I felt I knew how to live life properly and well. But as my disease wasted my body, it also demolished my knowledge of myself. As I have described, I no longer had confidence that I understood my past or what kind of person I had been in the past. Nor could I rely on past patterns of behavior and achievement as being reliable templates for my future. I was at a loss to know how to face the next day, much less how to build a future with family and friends. Since the whole context of my life and activity was redefined, I didn't know what were the appropriate emotional and behavioral responses to any given situation or relationship. Even if I had known how to respond to such unusual circumstances, I could not depend on my body, mind, or emotions to carry through with what I decided.

But the worst thing my disease did to me was to steal my God, at least the God I thought I had known in the past. I mourned for God. God was no longer my familiar friend, the one with whom I could share and worship. The God of my past was a healer and helper; God had saved me so many times! But, as I looked back, I began to wonder. Sudden remission of symptoms often occurs in MS. Had my remissions been coincidental to the faith and prayers of hundreds of people? Perhaps I had been mistaken to think that these remissions were any kind of sign that God was blessing a particular course of action in my life. They could very well be just the normal working of an insidious, capricious disease. As I reviewed it, the evidence for healing was completely ambiguous. It was quite possible I had had no healing at all. If this was the case, I was robbed of much of what I thought I knew of God and God's action in my life. Perhaps the spirit of Rising was all a sham, a bad joke, just a glittering dream that disappears as ephemeral health and strength evaporate into thin air. God became a stranger to me.

Furthermore, it appeared that God had never really intended me to have a special destiny, a mission, an overarching life task that I and I alone must fulfill. Had I been deceived all this time, believing I was so special? How could I have gone so wrong? How could God have let me go so wrong? Perhaps I was just a straw, blown by the winds of fate.

As my knowledge of myself, my world and my God failed, so did my answers to fundamental questions of being—the "why" questions. Previously I thought I knew the answer to "Why am I here?" I was here to serve God and my fellow human beings. But that answer seemed irrelevant because I was no longer able to serve in the ways I had served before, and I couldn't see any alternatives. The more outward, universal "why" questions which for thousands of years have given structure to the search for meaning seemed ethereal to me. I reduced them down to personal size: "Why me?" "Why now?" "Why should I go on?"

It was during this time that I stopped reading scripture. Every time my eye fell on a verse or passage, it seemed to speak of depression, judgment, or commands that I would never be able to keep. I also stopped praying. No words would come. No thoughts of my own could plumb the depths of my heart. I went to church but people there could not help me. No one, even in the healing churches, was healing multiple sclerosis. Worst of all, my song died. I did not sing again for nearly five years.

As human knowledge failed me and my own knowledge of myself failed, I moved into a kind of gray realm of "Unknowing." If I don't *know* and no other human beings *know*, who does know, and how can I find out?

I understood how Jeremiah could cry out at God in this way:

> *I am the one who has seen affliction under the rod of God's wrath; he has driven and brought me into darkness without any light; against me alone he turns his hand, again and again, all day long. He has made my flesh and my skin waste away, and broken my bones; he has besieged and enveloped me with bitterness and tribulation; he has made me sit in darkness like the dead of long ago. He has walled me about so that I cannot escape; he has put heavy chains on me; though I call and cry for help, he shuts out my prayer; he has blocked my ways with hewn stones, he has made my paths crooked... He has filled me with bitterness, he has sated me with wormwood. He has made my teeth grind on gravel, and made me cower in ashes; my soul is bereft of peace; I have forgotten what happiness is; so I say, "Gone is my glory, and all that I had hoped for from the Lord." (Jeremiah 3:1-18, portions)*

I could not remember that God had said in 1981 that I would climb high mountains, walk in dark valleys, and swim deep rivers. I certainly did not remember God's promise to be with me. It would not be until years later that I would realize that God had been with me the whole time, leading me to a deeper relationship with Godself than I could ever have imagined. At this time, I just lived the darkness—with no words, no song, no interpretation, no reason, no cause, and no comfort.

Seeking Who I AM

Seeking the Way

In 1987, the Fraleys moved into the condo upstairs from us at the time when my health was going downstairs. Diane was small-boned and olive skinned with short black hair and flashing, intelligent eyes. I could immediately tell she had a high-strung temperament commensurate with her Italian genes. The first day I met her we exchanged neighborly pleasantries and I learned that she was a qualitative market researcher. She specialized in doing focus group work for large companies, helping them learn critical information about their products and services and the ways they fit with people's lifestyles. She told me she was starting her own business and was in need of a writer to work with her on reports for companies such as Procter & Gamble and The Discovery Channel.

Market research? I never heard of it. The business world was as alien to me as Mars. Even so, I knew I could write, and I offered my services on a free-lance basis for some of her projects. The arrangement had a lot of advantages for both of us. Since she traveled a lot, it was convenient that I was on-site and quickly available when she needed me. I also brought creativity and skill to her fledgling company and was willing to build new skills. From my side, it was an opportunity to do interesting work and make some money without leaving the house. This was the beginning of a fourteen-year relationship that was rich and productive for both of us, stimulating us both to grow personally and professionally. Over the coming years we would do a great variety of cutting-edge research for Fortune 100 companies, all based on live interviews with individuals and groups.

I performed my market research work in the very small world of my sunroom, which overlooked Madison Park, a four-block-long residential park with an oval drive that encircled gardens and shaded lawns. Diane would go out around the country collecting data and bring it home to me. She was sensitive to my needs as a disabled person and helped me set up a work environment that eventually included hardwiring into her computer network. It was okay with her for me to arrange my time to accommodate needed rest periods. My job not only provided income to help us support the family, but, just as important, for the next fourteen years it provided an important link for me to the outside world, a way I could stay in touch and interact in hidden but meaningful ways. When I first started the job, however, all of that was an unknown future.

I went through the outward motions of each day, doing what I had to do. Inwardly, my soul was dark, and I felt dead. I did not know that darkness is the medium in which God does the most creative work. Genesis says that in the beginning darkness was upon the face of the deep and the Spirit of God moved upon the waters. Then God said, "Let there be light." The Apostle John says of Christ, "The light shines in the darkness, and the darkness did not overcome it." I would never have believed I was ripe for creation. The depths of my despair became the chaos on which the Holy Spirit would move to make me a new creation.

Previously, my spiritual eyes had been turned outward, seeking missions, causes, and actions that I could pursue with my energy and ideas that I could explore with my intellect. My prayers had been mostly "exterior" prayers, prayers that related primarily to the external world, God's action in it, and my relationship to it. Now my spiritual eyes began to turn inward. Without my realizing it, God began to give me tools and gifts to construct a new life and a new spirituality, a new way of seeing myself and my God. I can't say I appreciated them at the time. It really seemed I just didn't have any alternative.

One of the tools God gave me was meditation, a gift that can only be exercised when one is quiet for long enough to hear one's own thoughts and—perhaps—the thoughts of God. Meditation was completely foreign to my previous experience. Growing up and living most of my life in the fundamentalist/evangelical framework, I never came into contact with classical teachings or modes of meditation.

As a matter of fact, such practices were regarded as dangerous and as potentially leading one into demonic influence. I had no role models and no literature to draw on, no great examples of the blessed saints of the church to guide me. Nevertheless, I was on a classical path, even though I did not realize it at the time, reinventing the wheel that would help carry me to health.

There was no word that said, "Let there be light." There was no voice of revelation, no lightning. There was nothing I could recognize as divine action to set the elements whirling until I was reborn. God used the voice of a friend.

The phone rang. Millie said, "Anna, seek God."

I, who had told so many others to do the same thing, was at a loss for myself. "How?" I asked.

She said, "Read the Bible every day."

It seemed pedantic and too simple. But I could not shut out Millie's voice. She was too good a friend. I had said similar things to her in the past, and she had heard my voice. I responded to her command with what seemed to me at the time a pure act of will, even though my personal will was a small, beaten, impotent thing. Somewhere inside me was a spark of God longing to be kindled into flame. In the darkness, God began nurturing that tiny spark.

I sought God as best I could. I pretended I was one of my own hard-core rehab cases from the past, and I counseled myself. I tried to do what I told me. It was hard. I set myself a schedule to read the Bible before I started writing early in the morning. At one time I had read the Bible voraciously. Now I was lucky to put in five minutes at it. The words were dry and cold. As soon as I was finished reading, the words would fly right out of my head, and I would be depressed again, taking refuge in my work.

To combat disinterest, I began copying Bible verses on post-it notes and sticking them all around my computer, on my desk, my lamps, anything I was likely to glance at during the day. I put up encouraging verses, from the Psalms mostly. I listened to worshipful music to soften my hard heart. At the best of times, I felt like a weary soul in a dry, dry land.

One day God spoke to me in a dream:

I was taking a shortcut through a wood to avoid a long curve in the highway on which I was walking. I could see the far side of the sweeping curve through the trees and thought I could easily get back on it again before dark. On my way through the woods, I passed a tall dirt bank, and my attention was captured by a shiny object protruding from it. I stopped, slipped off my backpack, and scratched in the dirt, soon pulling out a silver knife. More scratching revealed another item close by the knife. I then began digging rapidly in the soft earth and soon pulled out a beautifully shaped silver teapot of intricate craftmanship, quite undamaged and only in need of a good polishing. My eye roved the bank, and I soon discovered more treasures. I set myself to pull them out and lay them beside my pack.

Before long, I had all the major pieces of a beautiful tea service in front of me. I was so busy I hardly noticed that a small group of people had pulled up folding lounge chairs on top of the bank and were casually watching me work, commenting on what I was finding.

My embarrassment caused me to stop and give them a tentative greeting. One of the older women only replied, "Why are you digging on my property?" Stunned, I found I had no answer.

"Well," she said, "I guess you know everything you find actually belongs to me."

I saw my work would go for nothing, but I replied feebly, "Suppose we split fifty-fifty, since I'm the one who found the stuff."

"Dig all you want," she said. "Nevertheless, what you find is mine. People dig around here all the time." She returned to her chair.

I looked at the pile lying next to me. Now it just seemed dirty and cheap. Then I noticed that daylight was vanishing. I couldn't see the highway through the woods any more. I heard a voice somewhere very close to me say, "Why are you digging here when there's a mother lode so nearby?"

While I don't often pay attention to dreams, this one seemed important. I prayed to understand what the highway was. Was it a course of action I should take that I had previously missed? Was it a mission I had wrongly interpreted? Was it some place I should have gone but didn't? When had I left the path? What had I done wrong? I thought if I knew what the highway was and where it went, I could get back on it. I could change my life to *do* what I should have been *doing* all the time. Then maybe I could be healed of my awful disease. The answer (the mother lode) was close to me, but I was unable to see it.

I had no quick answers to my questions. I laboriously followed my schedule of work and increased my Bible reading and prayer time until it was well established habit. Almost imperceptibly, my meditations began to feed me and lift my spirits, giving me strength to face each day. Depression began to disperse. While the light was not yet "shining" out of my darkness, at least a small spark began flickering somewhere inside me.

Finding "The Way"

I pondered the meaning of the dream for several weeks, although some of the meaning seemed immediately clear. I, who had always been so goal oriented, had lost all sense of direction and was spiritually wandering. I had stopped in my wanderings to dig up other people's treasures (other people's missions and causes) and was deceived for a while into thinking they were my own. Now they were lying uselessly at my feet. Obviously, I needed to get back on the highway, but I didn't know which way to turn because night had fallen. Most importantly, the dream spoke to me that there was a far greater treasure accessible to me, if only I looked in the right place.

The dream provided me with a story for meditation. I thought of myself in many different ways as being on a journey and seeking the path I should follow, just walking, seeking. Finally, one day when I was very quiet, I heard these words deep in my spirit: "I am the Way. Walk in the Way." I was surprised. I looked in the Bible at John 14:4-6 where Christ says to his disciples that they know where he is going and that they can also go there. Thomas responds, "We do not know where you are going. How can we know the way?" Christ answers, "I am the Way."

In Sunday school, from the time I was a babe, I had heard that Christ is "the Way." To me it had meant, for all practical purposes, "Follow Christ, do what he wants you to do, and go where he wants you to go. If you do that, you will "be what he wants you to be." The wrong headedness of this kind of thinking only dawned on me clearly now that I was no longer able to go or do. How could you *be* what he wants you to *be* if you could not follow him in the Way by *going* and *doing*? Did my inability to *go* and *do* mean that I could not follow Christ? Did it mean that I had no value as a person—or as a Christian? It was a difficult question for me. I wanted to scream, "No, no, no! I am still worth something, even when I can't *do* anything at all!" But I wasn't sure I was right. How can you *be* and not *do*? Do you have to *do* in order to *be*? I recalled the joke about the three philosophers discussing the meaning of existence, and all I could think of, cynically, was the Frank Sinatra answer: The meaning of life is "Do-be-do-be-do." It is all tied up together. How can you have one without the other? How can you sort it all out?

I came upon another scripture passage that clarified the problem somewhat. In Matthew 19, a rich ruler comes to Christ and asks him this question: "What must I do in order to be perfect?" The man is seeking acceptance in his own eyes and in the eyes of God in terms of things he could *do*. Christ asks whether he has kept the Ten Commandments, and he says he has kept them from the time he was a child. According to customary religious and human wisdom of his day, this man had *done* all that is possible for a human being to *do* to achieve the acceptance he coveted. Then Christ looks into his heart, sees his earnest desire, and calls him into a new dimension of living. He calls upon him to lay aside his current perception of self worth, defined in terms of doing what is right and expected in his religious framework. He says, "Sell all you have and give it to the poor and follow me."

For the rich ruler, this is a startling command. By saying, "Sell all you have and give it to the poor," Christ is calling him to go far beyond what the Jewish law demanded in giving one-tenth of his income. Christ opens the possibility of actions springing from a deeper place than obedience to "rules" and conformity to traditional religious precepts. By challenging him to give up all his attachments, Christ calls him from a framework of doing what is religiously right to a dimension of the heart—of *being* in relationship to God: "Follow me." The rich ruler, unable to accept the challenge, goes away sorrowfully. His investment in doing and having—and feeling righteous about it —is too great a sacrifice.

I puzzled over the story and how it might apply to me. It seemed that I, unlike the rich ruler, did not really have a choice about giving up *doing* as a foundation for my self-image. My doing was stripped from me without my permission by my disease. But I was hearing the same call, "Follow me." What did it mean for me to follow Christ in my disabled condition? How could you "walk in the Way" without going somewhere or doing something or having some destiny or mission in life? I couldn't imagine a life that was not mission-driven. Having a mission was the "right" and "righteous" thing to do for people in my religious circles. I was strongly attached to my missions, just as the rich young ruler was attached to his goods. My missions gave me self-identity and self worth in my context just as his "stuff" did for him. I was inexorably goal oriented. Nevertheless, I too was hearing the call, "Follow me."

I tried to think of a mental picture that would clarify the idea of following Christ without going anywhere or doing anything in particular. Perhaps a concrete image would help me implement into my life a very difficult concept. I tried out several pictures, but the one that seemed most effective was that of a narrow highway on which I was walking very closely behind Jesus. I had no idea of my final destination—I was just walking along in the present moment. My full attention was absorbed by the step I was currently taking. I did not look to either side of the road, nor did I look back at where I had come from. I was not allowed to look over Jesus' shoulder to see what lay ahead; my vision was fully consumed by the person of Jesus. My eyes could wander only from his head to his hands to his feet and observe his motion in front of me. That is all. I called this the "Picture of the Way."

Over a period of time, I found that this mental picture worked powerfully for me in several types of need. Sometimes I slipped into "future shock," a state in which I would contemplate my future as a disabled person. I worked all the angles, trying to figure out God's plan for me. I presupposed what God would do for me or in me and what I would do for God because I loved God and wanted so much to do something. This brought me nothing but grief. My health made it impossible for me to plan even what I would do today or tomorrow, much less next month or next year. The way I felt could depend on the weather. When I became anxious about the future, envisioning the Picture of the Way called me back to the present moment and helped me refocus my attention on the one secure place in the Universe.

Whenever I thought of the past and began to feel depressed because I was not the person I used to be, I brought the Picture of the Way into mind. I focused on Christ, immediately in front of me, and reminded myself that I could not live in the past and could not define myself in the same ways I did before my illness. If I did, I grieved for the old person I was before and I denigrated the worth of the person I was now. The Picture of the Way reminded me to keep my attention on the present and on the One who walks in front of me. It reminded me to live one step at a time and one day at a time.

When I became envious of active people around me and when I coveted energy and strength to do things that are exciting or pleasurable—or even just to engage in normal, daily routines—fixing my eyes on Jesus helped me center my whole being. It reminded me that I was not stagnant—I was going somewhere right now, in this present moment, behind a trustworthy guide. I could take advantage of the opportunities that presented themselves as I walked along each day, provided that I continued to "walk" in Jesus' footsteps.

When I had been walking behind Jesus in this way for some time, I realized something wonderful. When I was walking behind Christ, I was no longer in the woods, and I was no longer lost. Nor was I digging up other people's treasures. It seems that the simple act of shifting my gaze to Christ was having the amazing effect of moving me closer to him. Not only that. It was giving definition and direction to my life and was saving me from the encroaching darkness around me.

I did not know it, but I was learning a fundamental principle that would strengthen me through many years to come: If I could fix my eyes on Christ, I would never be lost. Since that was the case, I needed to learn how to gaze very steadily in his direction.

Being Who I Am

One morning, as I continued my extended meditation on the Picture of the Way, I realized I was looking at Christ's back, not at his face. Furthermore, I only visualized him—I didn't speak with him. Why wasn't I conversing with this person in front of me? Why couldn't I see his face? Were we friends? I needed a friend. Or was he a convenient, useful figment of my imagination? Did I have access to his presence as a friend? When I looked at my crippled body, I didn't feel worthy to have such a companion. All the theology in the world could testify to me that I was God's child, but my disability caused me to believe that there was an unforgivable, innate flaw in my person that kept me from an intimate relationship with the person in front of me. I could follow him, but not speak with him. Perhaps Christ had to be the one to initiate the conversation.

It was during this time that I began another exercise that I called "holy imagination." Holy imagination occurred when I turned all my inward eyes toward Christ and tried to look into him to see that which is only possible in the "abundantly far more" of God. If I were quiet enough and looked long enough, the Holy Spirit would open my eyes and my ears and my heart.

One day I read this verse in Hebrews 4:16: "Let us therefore come boldly unto the throne of grace, that we may obtain mercy, and find grace to help in time of need." I read Hebrews 10:19, which says: "Having boldness to enter the holiest place . . ." I tried using holy imagining to envision myself coming boldly into God's presence; I tried to envision myself seeing Christ's face. It was very difficult. I spent some weeks during my early morning meditations turning my gaze toward Christ and not seeing anything. I tried out several mental pictures to help me envision what it would be like to boldly enter God's presence. I started with a picture of the ancient Hebrew tabernacle, which I had studied in great detail. I pictured God's presence as being in the holy of holies, the innermost sanctum of the Hebrew place of worship. In the ancient tabernacle there were three courts, an outer one where sacrifices were offered, a holy place where only priests could go, and an inner sanctum called the holy of holies, in which the Lord's presence resided between two cherubim above the Ark of the Covenant. I knew that in the Old Testament the rituals allowed only the high priest to enter the holy of holies once a year, but I tried to envision myself coming boldly in and having free access, as the New Testament declares we have access to God through Christ. In keeping with the ancient times of the tabernacle, and with the need for boldness, I pictured myself as a valiant warrior dressed for battle, perhaps looking like King David. I tried to imagine how I would feel, how I would act, and how Christ would respond to my entry into the holy place. I tried to imagine the expression on my face and the tone of his voice when Christ would speak to me. Would it be a voice of awe? Would there be smoke and thunder? Would I fall on my face in astonishment?

My meditation was suddenly interrupted with recognition of the complete absurdity of the scene I had just drawn for myself. I had been thinking, "How will *he* (the warrior) act? How will *he* feel? What will the Lord say to *him*?" In astonishment, I said to myself, "I am not *he*. I am not *male*! I am *female*. Why do I see a *male* warrior?"

The longer I looked at my mental picture, the more ridiculous and the more revealing it became. I am not a male, and I am certainly not a warrior! Why am I dressing myself up in the 3000-year-old garb of the opposite sex with a temperament and character and culture wholly different from my own? It was all wrong.

I flashed another image on the screen of my mind. I looked down at myself in the holy of holies and saw myself as a female. I gave myself a series of quick costume changes. First, I dressed myself in biblical robes. It didn't work. I was living in 1989, A.D., not 1000 B.C. I tried a series of modern outfits. What would be right to wear to enter the presence of the Lord of the Universe? A business suit? I don't go to the office any more. An evening gown? Too formal—when did I last wear one? A Sunday dress? A pant suit?

Finally I flipped the right slide into my mental projector. I caught my breath, then burst into tears when I looked down at myself. I had on a turquoise sweat suit and a big, oversized pair of down slippers to keep my feet warm. I wasn't striding boldly into the holy of holies; I was riding my electric scooter into my own sunroom!

"Oh, dear God," I thought. "I am myself!"

Who I Am As Myself

The series of images I had created about myself entering God's presence made me realize what a distorted, unhealthy perception I had of myself as a disabled person. I could more easily imagine myself as a 3000-year-old male warrior than as my very own self in God's presence. The corollary of this was that I couldn't imagine God receiving me into God's presence as a disabled person. Separation from human companionship produces a corresponding spiritual delusion.

But that wasn't all. The imaging process I started had a momentum and life of its own, and it continued evolving intermittently over several weeks. As time passed, I found myself wondering whether there was handicap access to this room where God was. Were there steps, or was there a ramp? These questions may have occurred to me because my disciplined habits of meditation had given me the unconscious impression that each day I was going in and out of God's presence when I began and ended my meditation time. I would wake up at 5:30 A.M., dress, eat breakfast, do a few exercises, and go to my office. Then I would "enter God's presence," read scripture for a while, listen to music and pray. Then I would "exit" to start my work.

I thought about it. I was entering God's presence for a few minutes and then leaving for the rest of the day. What a silly idea. Why would I want to leave? Why couldn't I stay there and enjoy the company, even while I was working? But this raised a new problem. How could I stay in God's presence? I pictured myself setting up camp in the holy place, putting down a sleeping bag and pushing the scooter out of the way. I resisted temptations to envision myself as suddenly and dramatically healed and skipping blithely out the door. No, I decided, I am here "just as I am, without one plea." I even sang the song "Just as I Am" to emphasize the point. I reminded myself throughout the day, each day, that I was continually in God's presence. After a while I began to accept that it was true, although the mundane space of my office suggested no outward evidence and I experienced no inner glory. The disciplined practice seemed to create an inner affirmation.

Holy imagining carried me forward. Pretty soon I got tired of the scenery in that small, enclosed space into which I had locked God and myself. The holy place I had designed in my mind was too narrow and confining to be interesting for very long. I wasn't sure what to do or say beyond the humdrum daily patter of, "Good morning, God, how are you today, it's good to have you here. I look forward to hanging out with you while I do my work." It seemed a bit too pedantic. Think about it. What would *you* say to the Lord of the Universe if you were stuck with him or it or her or whatever for twenty-four hours a day? It wasn't very personal. It was just an imagined presence, without form, warmth, personality, potency.

This way of viewing the relationship was perhaps a partial result of the fact that I spent almost all of my time in one room of the house, my sunroom-office. I perceived myself as static, rooted to one little spot, and I pulled God in around me, making God the size of my world. Not very many people came and went in this world. It was a little boring. And my imagined Presence wasn't doing much except being there.

Eventually, I realized that my small human context was limiting my conception of God, and I felt I must intentionally expand my perception, allowing God to fill larger and larger space so that no matter where I am or what I am doing God will be there, present with me. I practiced amplifying my idea of God. I tried to think of God being everywhere, filling more and more of what I know, beginning with smaller places and expanding out into larger and larger unknown spaces. I visualized in some detail what it would be like with God in our home, in our residential park, in the city of Chicago, in the United States, in the whole world. And then, because Don is an astronomer, I pictured God as filling the universe and dwelling around and through all planets, stars, pulsars, galaxies, all interstellar space, and beyond in other universes besides our own. I pictured God's freedom of movement, only a divine thought making God instantly present anywhere and everywhere. I pictured God in power, creating worlds from nothing. I imagined myself with God, watching supernovae explode, riding through black holes, transcending time and space. I repeated various aspects of this exercise many times as an opening to my meditations in order to allow God to be as big as possible in my thoughts.

In the midst of these meditations one morning, I was startled by a sudden change in vision, as though my spiritual channels were changed without permission. Incredibly, the omnipotence, the glory, the omnipresence I had been imagining was suddenly shrunk horribly down to small human size, deflated like a popped balloon. I looked up to see a poor fellow standing on a dusty road with his back to me. He slowly turned around. I looked at his head, his hands, his feet. They were scarred. It was Jesus. I was seeing him face to face.

In those days nothing registered quickly with me. I wasn't sure how to deal with what I had just seen, so I simply put my Bible away and went to work on my market research. Each day, however, I "picked up" the mental picture where I had left it and took another look.

One day I picked it up, looked at this Jesus, who was now looking back at me, and I said, "I see, Jesus, that you are a disabled person."

"Yes," he replied, and smiled.

When those of us who are handicapped get together, we often swap stories of what it is like to try to get a along in the outer world:

> *"I don't know what they were thinking about when they built that so-called accessible building. There's a one-and-a-half-inch step before you can get to the ramp. How will I get my electric wheelchair up that!"*
>
> *"The other day I was returning to my van in my wheelchair, and this SUV had parked in the striped side zone so I couldn't get in my car! It was 25 degrees and windy and I had to wait for him to return. He didn't even apologize."*

Then after those types of stories, we may get around to sharing the deeper struggles, stories of disappointment, loss of jobs, divorce, isolation, the death of a friend who died from your own disease. You always know when the other person has been there. She will look you in the eye and listen carefully, nodding her head. "Mmhmm. That's the way it is. Yeah." Then there's a pause and a deep breath. There is a feeling of being purged, cleansed, renewed, because someone else has listened and understood. You are not alone. Life can go on.

In my holy imagining, Jesus and I "swapped stories." I had heard sermons all my life about Christ suffering on the cross. I remember sitting on a hard pew as a little child, weeping my eyes out while the preacher passionately described the gruesome details of his crucifixion: "And the nails pierced his hands and feet and ripped into his flesh as his body hung there. His rib cage was hyper extended so he could barely draw a breath, and a horrible thirst seized him. Jesus said, 'I thirst.'" As the preacher grew more passionate, I recall weeping shamelessly, wiping my little nose on my sleeve and on the skirt of my Sunday dress. The worst of all was when the preacher said in a heart-rending crescendo, "And just before he died, he said, 'My God, my God, why hast thou forsaken me!' He died alone! And he did it for you!" The preacher boomed, "It was your sins that nailed him there!" I trembled and wept at the horror. The preacher always concluded such sermons with an admonition to confess our sins, repent and live for Jesus. I did. I confessed and repented of any lie I had ever told or any trick I had ever played on my sisters or on the family dog. I confessed leaving a strip of grass uncut while mowing the lawn and not feeding my pet rabbit. I even confessed things I thought about but didn't do. I confessed for everyone who ever did anything bad to me. I confessed all the things I might do in the future! I didn't want Jesus to suffer any more because of me!

Somehow, through all the years when I was a healthy person, I focused on my responsibility as a sinner when I heard such sermons. Christ's pain was a stimulus for me to feel the guilt of sin and to repent. Now, as a handicapped person who was sitting in Jesus' Presence, I quieted my own feelings and opened my heart to listen to his side of the story. How did he feel as a disabled person? I was drawn to that passage we heard over and over again when someone preached about the crucifixion, the one in Isaiah 53, the one about the suffering servant. It says, "He was wounded for our transgressions, bruised for our iniquities . . . He was cut off out of the land of the living, stricken for the transgression of my people." That was the sin and guilt part that required me to repent. But now it seemed Jesus was speaking in first person, not in the third person of the text. He was saying to me as I sat there with him, "I had no form or majesty that anyone should look at me. Nothing in my appearance would make anyone desire me. I was despised and rejected. I suffered, and I knew what it was like to be weak and sick. People hid their faces from me. I was crushed with pain. In my anguish, it was so dark I wondered if I would ever see the light."

As I heard him tell his story, I listened quietly and the tears came again. Not tears of guilt but tears of sharing. I looked deep into his eyes. Slowly, I nodded my head. "Mmhmm. Yes, that's the way it is." I knew he had been there.

Then he told me the deeper story, the life story, the story of how the dynamic energy of God was incarcerated in the prison of a frail human body. How strange it was to have to rest his physical body when his whole being cried out to work without ceasing, healing and preaching God's reign! The divine mind had to function in the confines of a human brain. His movement was restricted to the feeble power of human muscles, and his vision to the human eye. How strange it was to be dependant on others for food, shelter, and companionship. Even his emotions were captive to his human nature, and he prayed to avoid the worst of human realities, death.

"Oh dear God," I thought as I listened, "he too struggled with the dilemma of being a spiritual person in a human body. He too struggled with doing and being, mission and meaning, and it was all because he chose to take on human form." The familiar scripture in Philippians 2:6-8 came to life for me in a new way:

> *Though he was in the form of God, [he] did not regard equality with God as something to be exploited, but emptied himself, taking the form of a slave, being born in human likeness. And being found in human form, he humbled himself and became obedient to the point of death—even death on a cross. (NRSV)*

Christ took human form. I thought about it. If someone else had my disabilities and I were a healthy person, would I be willing to trade places, knowing what I know now? Christ had made that choice. He became trapped, handicapped, by a human body in order to show his love. Then he endured the ultimate insult, a tortured, disfiguring death.

I looked in amazement at this Christ. Yes, he was there. Yes, he understood. Yes, I knew that Jesus is like me. We shared deeply the profound mystery of life, of what it is like to dwell in a human body. I felt purged, cleansed, renewed. I was not alone. Life could go on.

I stayed in his presence, the presence of the Disabled One. The longer I was there the more I saw with my inward eyes that Jesus' human weakness was the very basis and fundamental principle of his power. Jesus' human disabilities, all of his human likeness, constituted no barrier whatever to his receiving the full love of God or to his full performance of the will of God. God has performed his greatest act of love through the broken, imperfect, crucified, human body of Jesus. God's love, as scripture says, has been made perfect in weakness; God's power has come to full strength in imperfection. This, I saw, is the meaning of the Incarnation, of Christ coming to dwell in a human body. Christ came in a body like ours to show that God's power and love can triumph over every human weakness. It is in this human body that we must do all of our work here on this earth, that we must show forth the power of God's love, no matter how weak and broken the body is.

I realized I could boldly enter and remain in God's presence because Christ is like me and fully understands me, even with all my disabilities, perhaps even because of my disabilities. He invites me to be there and receives me in love and mercy. His greatest act of love is becoming like me, becoming—yes—disabled. Seeing this love of Christ caused me to see myself in a different light too. I asked myself, "Who am I when I am with Christ?" The answer came back, "I am loved."

Being Empty and Full

Before I opened my eyes, I heard the snow shovel scraping on the sidewalk outside. "So it snowed last night," I thought. I wondered how much. I sat on the edge of the bed and looked out between the slats of the Venetian blinds. Sure enough, Denny, the building custodian, was outside shoveling, and it looked like the snow was four or five inches deep and still coming down. "Okay, so no church for me today." When there was snow on the ground, it was a major mess to get me anywhere. First, it was getting through two doors of the narrow little elevator, then through two heavy exterior doors, then through the snow to the car, packing up the chair with the spokes full of snow, getting the trunk full of melted water— it just wasn't worth the hassle. By the time I got to church I'd be worn out with it anyway. I roused the rest of the family and got them started.

There was the usual Sunday morning hubbub.

"I can't find my socks!"

"They're on the dryer." I knew they were there because Dorothy had sorted them on Friday and had laughingly given me the tally. There were 96 socks and 32 of them had no matches!

"I can't find Alice." Alice was Jeremy's guinea pig, and, being a bright little pig, she always hid under beds to avoid being put in her cage.

"You have to find her before you go to church. She'll pee all over the rug."

"Somebody ate all my Captain Crunch!"

"Eat Raisin Bran."

"Do I have to wear a button shirt? Mine is not ironed."

Amidst the family clatter, I finally rolled into the dining room for my own breakfast. Don put my cereal bowl on the table for me, but with all the activity, he forgot to get me a spoon. I pushed away from the table and headed through the archway into the kitchen, meeting him coming the other direction. We didn't fit through the door together, and he was in a hurry. "So what do you need?" His voice sounded edgy.

"I just need a spoon, that's all."

"Well, why didn't you ask for one?"

"I just thought I'd get it myself." He was already on the way, grabbing a spoon from the drawer and a half gallon of milk from the fridge, then wheeling me back around into the dining room and placing me at the table.

"Anything else?" he asked.

"I need that plastic cup with the handle." I had trouble grasping a regular glass, but I disliked causing him trouble. Shortly the cup appeared with tea in it. "Thanks." He bent down to give me a kiss and a hug. "Sorry I was so short," he said. I patted his hand.

Sudden quiet replaced the morning roar as the family exited for church. I sat at the table for a few moments, finishing my tea and thinking about the morning that stretched before me. Then I slowly wheeled myself into my office. I looked out at the snow-laden branches of the oak outside my window, wondering how the squirrels were faring in the deep snow. I had watched them industriously gathering acorns throughout the fall, and I suspected that there was a deep storehouse behind that hole that was nearly at my eye level. As I watched, a gray squirrel poked her head out and then emerged, sniffing the air and whisking the branch free of snow with her tail. I sat there watching for a moment, wondering what life would be like inside that hole. Then the squirrel darted back in and disappeared from my sight, entering a world known only by squirrels. I pulled back into my own small space of the sunroom.

Being alone on Sunday morning highlighted my inability to share in community and serve as others do. I felt shut in. I felt empty. I closed my eyes and sat there quietly for a while until I could begin my meditation. Slowly I began to visualize myself in God's presence, talking with Christ. I presented myself to him. "See?" I said, in a rather accusatory tone. "I am sad. I have come empty. I have no gift for you."

"Is that so?" he said. "What would you like to give me?"

"Jesus," I said, "here I am sitting here by myself, everyone is gone—

I want to *do* something for you. I want to give you some service of love, some genuine, unique response to your love for me. I want to do something special for you, and my body won't let me."

"Really? Very well. You may give me the most precious gift of all. It is a service that will satisfy us both."

"Yes, Lord. Tell me what it is."

I waited, hoping to hear the words I had longed to hear all my life, the words that would tell me what I could *do* for him, the words that would reveal my own special mission for God, the words that would tell me how to express my love, perhaps the words of healing that would empower me to do his will.

"You have brought it with you. Give me your emptiness."

First I was shocked, then disappointed. Nothing at all. That's what I'd brought, nothing at all, and now he was saying he wanted me to give him *nothing*. How could *nothing at all* satisfy the Lord of the universe? How could *nothing at all* satisfy me? Sometimes in this sort of dialogue I got the feeling I must be fabricating the whole scene, especially when I didn't really want to hear what was being said. I was ready to do a rewind/erase on the conversation, but I paused for a moment as Jesus seemed to ask another question:

"How big am I?" Jesus asked.

I paused for a moment. It was an interesting question, one I had been meditating on for some time. "You fill all the universe and more," I replied slowly, and was about to reiterate the planet-stars-interstellar-space routine that had become a part of my morning litany.

"Not all of it," interrupted Jesus, raising his eyebrows.

I'm not a stupid person. It only took me a moment to catch on. I caught a glimpse of the void in myself, the lacuna that was my innermost being, the only place in the Universe I had not thought of asking Jesus to fill. The view into my own empty space was dizzying. Jesus was asking me to give it to him. I took the step: "Fill me, Lord."

"Yes. Thank you for your gift," he replied.

I remained quiet for some time, but when my mind was quite

blank for a while, I turned to other things, some singing, some reading. I knew I would discover more about this encounter in God's time. The morning passed.

In the following days I reflected on the conversation about emptiness. This whole situation was somewhat amusing. This was a permutation of the old dilemma, "What do you give the man or woman who has everything?" What do you give the infinite God who has everything? The answer: more space, my own personal space, the space over which I have control, my inner space.

I laughed, then I cried at my foolishness. I wanted to give and do, for God and others—and myself—out of my emptiness, out of my dislike—even my hatred of myself. Jesus was right. The void was there, awesome, desolate, forsaken. Yes, I was in the presence of God, and I was experiencing, at least on the surface, God's love for me. But there was something yet lacking for this love to become active in me. There was some missing catalyst needed to act on the inert elements that composed my heart and soul. What was the missing agent that would set off the desired chain reaction that would change me, change my life, and make me usable, make me capable of *doing* something for God, *heal me!*?

My devotional diary from this time shows an initial burst of enthusiasm at the prospect of being filled by Christ. I had been filled before. In 1972 my baptism of the Holy Spirit had been mighty and accompanied by powerful, overwhelming signs, physical, as well as spiritual. These signs had lasted over a long period of time and had genuinely changed and enriched my life and the lives of others. I reveled in the new possibilities. I prepared myself to receive. Jesus wanted to fill me anew. I had given him permission. How would it happen? When would it happen? How would it change me? Would I be healed when I was filled?

I concentrated on being open to all possibilities. I reminded myself of the void that needed filling and of God's power to fill it. I pictured the void, if one can do so. I envisioned myself as an empty clay vessel, waiting to be filled with wine, as Jesus had done miraculously at Cana. I pictured myself as a desert and imagined water springing up suddenly to water me and cause me to bloom. I wandered in the wilderness in my thoughts, and, like the ancient Israelites, I dug for water with a stick in the sand and sang, "Spring up, O well!" I sought shelter from the blazing sun in the shadow of a rock from which came oil and water. I was the woman at the well, Jesus offering me a well of water springing up to eternal life. I was the cripple at the pool of Bethesda, waiting for the water to move. I was in the crowd when Jesus, on the great day of the feast, shouted, "If anyone thirsts, let her come to me and drink. She that believes on me, as the scripture has said, out of her belly shall flow rivers of living water." I relived my trip to Israel, and, closing my eyes, I felt the water of the spring of Gihon in Jerusalem, flowing through the underground tunnel and rushing over my body, deeper and deeper, up to my neck as I waded through its cool, ancient streams.

Time passed. My pictures were not real. My visualizations came to nothing. My meditations produced no sudden revelations, no deep insights, no miracles of healing, no sense of the fullness of the Holy Spirit. After some weeks of offering myself for filling, I seemed emptier than ever. By meditating on the void within, it had become more real, my view into the emptiness more vertiginous.

It finally occurred to me that perhaps I was the victim of some joke of perspective. Perhaps I was a figure in an Escher lithograph, walking perfectly logically upside down or horizontally to the floor. Perhaps I was looking at a Gestalt and seeing the devil instead of the beautiful woman. Perhaps I was an outsider in a club of mathematicians that had turned a circle inside out and I hadn't caught the significance. Perhaps I needed to look at everything from a different angle.

I focused my inner eyes deeper into the One who knows me and the One whom I want to know so much but cannot know with any of my own natural abilities. As I became very quiet, I saw again the picture of Christ on the Way. I had left him there at the time he promised to fill me, and, apparently, I had gone off on my own little circular side trail. He was still there, quietly waiting for me, a quizzical expression on his face.

"What went wrong?" I asked.

"Nothing. I am here."

"You said you wanted to fill me. Why didn't you?"

"I did."

"With what, Lord?"

"Not with *what*. With *myself*."

I sat quietly for a moment, thinking. Then, slowly I said shamefully, "I don't think I recognized you."

"No, you didn't."

"Why, Lord?" I asked, crestfallen.

"Anna," he said very gently, "when you looked inside yourself, you saw emptiness and you thought it was your own. You didn't know you were seeing me.

"What do you mean, Lord?"

Anna, don't you remember, that when I became a human, I emptied myself?"

Hmm. I thought back to the Philippians 2 passage on which I had been meditating recently:

> *Though he was in the form of God, [he] did not regard equality with God as something to be exploited, but emptied himself, taking the form of a slave, being born in human likeness. And being found in human form, he humbled himself and became obedient to the point of death—even death on a cross. (NRSV)*

I had been impressed that when Christ became a human he had emptied himself in love for *me*. I had not focused on the remarkable statement that he *emptied himself*.

"You emptied yourself... I think I always thought of you as being full—full of love."

"That's right. I am."

"But you say you are empty."

"Yes."

There was a long pause. "Help me, Lord."

"Anna, when I poured myself out, I became empty. When one gives everything in love, there is nothing left of self. There is emptiness. Perfect love is perfect emptiness."

I was speechless. It wasn't that I was unfamiliar with the theological idea that Jesus poured out his nature as God. But this was not theological. It was personal, intimate, concrete emptiness that was confronting me. The emptiness of selfless love. Jesus was saying this kind of love was filling me. What an outrageous thought.

"How, can that be, Lord? I do not have this in me. I could never have this in me."

"No, you don't, and you can't have it of yourself. But I have it, and I am in you."

It took a long time for this to register. Slowly, I tried to articulate the shadows of my thoughts. "I looked inside myself and saw emptiness and thought it was my own, but it was really yours?"

As you become more of who I AM, I become more of who YOU ARE.

I needed to meditate on this for a long time. I had come to the Lord believing I was empty and Christ had shown me that I am full. But it was not fullness in the sense I wanted, requested, or expected. I had really been wanting the power to express my love, especially through actions and overt service. I had wanted to be full of *doings*. But Christ had very stubbornly bypassed my desires and requests and had insisted on filling me with a gift of his own choice—himself. And it wasn't the Christ I had known in the past. It was a Christ who was confronting me with his own radical emptiness and saying that emptiness is the fullness of love.

The confrontation not only demanded that I see Jesus differently but that I change my view of myself. If Christ was in me and filling me—even in my weak, impotent, disabled condition, I could no longer feel sorry for myself because of my suffering; I could no longer complain about my emptiness and my inability to *do*; I could no longer hate myself and wallow in guilt. Christ was not shrinking from me. He was entering deeply and profoundly into my emptiness and even, it seemed, inviting me to share in his own, to become his own. He was compelling a transformation in my perception of Who He Is and showing me Who I Am.

There was something about being seriously disabled that made me desire affirmation not only from myself, my loved ones and from all human beings. I wanted to find myself at one, at peace with the Universe itself, with Christ, with the Creator of the Universe! An earthquake was moving in me, irrevocable, unstoppable. Deep insights were forming in the tectonic plates of my innermost being, out of my conscious sight and understanding. In coming years, they would come up to the surface and I would see from ever-new perspectives the mystery of creation and re-creation, of birth and rebirth, of death and resurrection. The void, the chaos, the darkness, the stillness is the medium in which the Spirit moves and into which God speaks the words, "Let there be light." Darkness is the medium through which God created the world and through which God would re-create me. What seems to be death is the condition in which life rises and begins again. Emptiness is the fullness of God's possibilities.

Meeting the "I AM"

After several months of training and focusing my thoughts and practicing the discipline of The Picture of the Way, I realized that my whole view of life was changing. I was concentrating less on where I was going and what I was doing and was becoming more and more aware of the Presence who was with me. In the words "I am the Way," which I called frequently to mind, the word "Way" became less and less important. The words "I AM" began to vibrate with life, like strings untouched for too long in the depths of my spirit. I remembered what I had known for a very long time but in the press of suffering had forgotten: God's name is Yahweh, or "I AM." Yahweh is the God who *is*, the God of Being. This was the revelation God gave to the patriarchs. When Moses wanted to know God's name, God said "I AM THAT I AM," a way of saying "I AM the fullness of being, everything that has been, everything that is and everything that will be." Throughout the recorded history of Israel, God would, at various times, connect the name I AM with a divine quality that addressed human need, such as I AM Your Provider, I AM Your Healer, I AM Your Righteousness, I AM Your Strength. When God's people called on a particular name, God would bring a powerful manifestation of it into their lives. Some of the greatest stories of scripture are associated with these names of God. For example, the name I AM Peace was revealed to Gideon during the tribulation of a war with the Midianites, one of Israel's most fierce enemies. The name disclosed the possibility of having "peace that passes understanding" in the midst of great distress. The name empowered Gideon to turn to God for strength to defeat his enemies.

Christ used the I AM name in his ministry, making powerful I AM statements such as "I AM the Way," "I AM the Light of the World:" "I AM the Bread of Life;" "I AM the Door;" "I AM the Good Shepherd, and even "I AM the Resurrection and the Life." By saying, "I AM" in this way he was identifying himself with God in such a powerful way that those in the religious establishment regarded it blasphemous, a claim of actually being God. Such statements, coupled with Christ's blatant disregard for Jewish law and tradition eventually led to his crucifixion.

In the past I had learned that calling on a specific I AM name of God or Christ had great power to produce faith and bring a particular attribute of the divine nature into manifestation in my life. Unfortunately, the long years of illness and suffering had caused me to forget the power that was available and had blunted my ability to reach out for it. I had been bitter and angry about the past; I had been fearful of the future; I had loathed the pain and loneliness of the present.

But now I was experiencing more peace. Being in the presence of the I AM was having the remarkable effect of healing time. The past and the future were shrinking to narrower dimensions, gradually becoming places too small for escape, too thin in which to hide. The more I was in the Presence, the more I was able to live in the present. I was stirred to a new awareness that I could call on I AM and that the power of I AM could be manifest in my life right now. Even more, I came to greater awareness that I could not only call on I AM but that I am made in the image of God and that I am, therefore, a human *being*. It is my nature not just to *do* but also to *be*. I AM is fundamentally at the core of my being; therefore, to call on I AM is to call my own most powerful, dynamic essence into manifestation in my life.

Meeting the I AM who is God and the I AM who is also in some mysterious way myself is an experience of the Present but not of a single day. The revelation of what it would mean to me would begin unfolding in my innermost being and for many years to come I would be exploring what it means to become all I can BE, all I AM.

A "Rising" Manifesto

A Mountaintop Experience

Apache Point Observatory, located in the Sacramento Mountains of New Mexico, is now a bustling scientific center with two of the world's great telescopes peering out into space and collecting data that is radically changing our view of the Universe. In the late 1980's it was a quiet site in the national forest, just beginning to come to life. Don, as Founding Director of the Observatory, was giving birth to a cutting-edge, 3.5-meter, remotely-controlled telescope, and he needed to be on site to make sure the project was off to a good start. We arrived at Apache Point in the summer of 1989 to stay for a month, but Don soon concluded that he needed to be there for a full year to oversee the mirror installation and the first operations of the telescope. From the Chicago end I would never have considered the possibility because of the massive task of getting the whole family ready to move for a year. But from the New Mexico end it looked appealing.

Amazingly, the pieces fell together to make it happen. Yes, we could rent our cottage for a year; yes, the astronomy department at Chicago would approve Don's leave. I made all the arrangements for renting our Chicago condo by telephone and made long lists of things we needed and things that had to be done when Don went back to Chicago for a week. I was doing pretty well physically, enjoying a reprieve during which I was able to walk short distances. We enrolled the boys in school in Cloudcroft, a mountain village about sixteen miles from the observatory, assembled odds and ends of furnishings for our cottage and settled in.

We lived in Sunspot, a tiny community of about fifty people around the bend from Apache Point. Located at an altitude of 9200 feet at the end of a highway in a national forest, Sunspot's reason for existence is to service the National Solar Observatory, a research facility for studying the Sun, including the "sunspots" that give the community its name. Cloudcroft is the nearest outpost where one can pick up a gallon of milk, and it is thirty-six miles to the nearest good grocery shopping in Alamagordo. Sunspot and Apache Point boast spectacular, expansive views down onto the sparkling White Sands in the Tularosa Valley, one mile below. The air is clear, the skies blue, and the forests full of wildlife. This place alone is beautiful enough to earn New Mexico its designation as the "Land of Enchantment."

We settled into our little home and put the kids in school, and life began to assume a tranquil pace quite different from that of the bustling city from which we had come. The big events in Sunspot were volleyball games on Thursdays and movies on Friday nights in the community center. On Saturdays the family always went down the mountain for groceries because our apartment-size fridge wouldn't hold enough food for our hungry troops. In between, my time was my own. It was a perfect place to stop, look back, and reconsider all that had happened to me in the previous years. It was here in this place of natural beauty and vision that I had a mountaintop experience. My reflections resulted in development of a "Rising Manifesto" that would undergird me as I experienced the next few years of even greater pain and suffering. Still more important, the core principles I developed during this time would pave the way for amazing healing on the other side of that suffering.

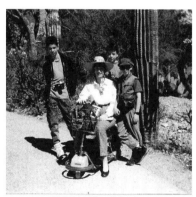

*1989 in New Mexico:
A rare photo of me in my scooter,
with three of our sons, Maurice,
Chandler, and Jeremy.*

Snowstorm

Alamogordo is a modest-sized town on the desert one mile in altitude below Apache Point. It borders on the White Sands, a gleaming stretch of gypsum sand dunes formed by minerals that have leached out of the mountains for thousands of years and have piled up in big mounds in the Tularosa valley. The dunes are a natural wonder, the best "beach" in the world, except, of course, there is no water. "Alamo" is the gateway to the White Sands Missile Range, which stretches for miles along the valley floor and includes the test site where the first atomic bomb was detonated.

I sometimes went down the mountain to Alamo to use the Public Library. I enjoyed the scenic drive, even though some parts of it were quite precipitous and full of blind S-curves. There was usually little traffic, but it was possible to get stuck behind a slow-moving lumber truck and be forced to follow it all the way up or down, whichever way I was traveling. I noticed a strange feature of the mountain geology and climate. Down in Alamo there are palm trees, and in the summer it's very hot. In the winter the temperature rarely drops below freezing. A few miles up the mountain there is a tunnel that seems to mark a sudden change in the terrain and climate. On the lower end it is rocky, brown and dry. When one emerges on the upper end, there is verdant green countryside, spotted with cherry and apple orchards, almost a little paradise. Farther up, the pine forest begins, interspersed with aspen.

I was driving up the mountain late on a winter's day, knowing I would finish the trip after sunset. I was still a greenhorn about mountain weather, so I found it fascinating when a thunderstorm roared through Alamo that afternoon, dumping cup-sized raindrops and hail the size of ping-pong balls. As I headed home there were breaks in the clouds, but the air seemed heavy and thick. I steered the big blue Oldsmobile station wagon up the hill toward the tunnel, thinking about the turkey dinner Don would be fixing that evening. A little shower spattered the windshield here and there, but nothing serious. Then I came to the tunnel. The darkness surrounded me, and I looked for the dim light at the other end. As I pulled out on the upper side, I was surprised that the sprinkles of rain had become snow and that it was beginning to stick to the ground. How could there be such a big change in such a short time! I continued up the mountain to Cloudcroft, the little village sixteen miles below Sunspot and the last outpost of civilization before I reached home. From Cloudcroft to Sunspot there were a few isolated homesteads, but most of them were only occupied in the summer. I noticed there was some ice under the snow as I pulled into the Cloudcroft Inn to call Don. "Hi, Lover," I said. "I'm in Cloudcroft, and it's snowing, but Bert says he thinks it may stop soon, so I'm going to head on up there."

"You can stay the night at the motel if you want to," he said. I felt Don was always being overprotective. He was always pointing out that if I had trouble I wouldn't be able to walk for help. Right. Well, I had driven in plenty of snow before, and this didn't seem that bad. "Nah!" I said. It's no big deal, I'll be fine." I hung up and headed for the car.

While I was inside the Inn, another inch of snow had fallen on the windshield. I took the brush off the seat and whisked off the side windows and my side of the windshield. After shaking off my shoes, I closed the car door and fastened my seat belt. Then I turned the key, started the engine and set the windshield wipers in motion. The snow was heavy and wet, and the wipers scooped it slowly across the window with a muffled whoosh. I switched on the headlights, and as I turned onto the road, I noticed there was no traffic. The night was silent and dark, except for the large snowflakes blowing across my headlights.

I began the ascent, rounding the cliff below the Lodge and making for the turn that would take me to Sunspot. I turned right and moved on up into the forest. The pine trees, already loaded with snow, loomed like great white spectres on either side of the road. In an imaginary conversation with Don, I was saying, "I'm doing fine, just fine, thank you. No sweat."

Two or three miles later, the road was getting steep and I was headed into that part of the route where there was a series of S-curves. Many of them had a ditch and a steep cliff on one side and a sheer drop-off on the other. I was now moving slowly, and I began to feel anxious. The snow was not letting up at all. As a matter of fact, it was coming down harder and heavier than ever. I took the center of the road because I wasn't sure where the edges were. I thought perhaps I should turn around and go back, but as I assessed my situation, I realized I was at the point of no return as far as safety was concerned. The way back down the mountain would be just as hazardous as going forward. Besides, there were now no side roads where I could make the turnaround. The windshield wipers were working hard and slow to keep the snow clear. Whoosh! Whoosh!

The higher I climbed, the deeper the snow became, and I could now feel that there was a layer of ice underneath. Soon I was going forward at a crawl. I took my foot off the gas, and to my horror I felt the car slide backward down the mountain, pulled by the weight of gravity across the slippery ice. The tires didn't have enough tread to hold it to the road. That wasn't the worst of it though. At that point the road was graded toward the drop-off, and as the car slid back it also slipped sideways toward the precipice. I caught my breath, realizing I had to keep up a certain momentum or the weight of the car could take me down and slide me right off into darkness below. Suddenly my body tensed all over as I pictured the car plunging down and landing in the forest, 150 feet straight down, covered with snow and lost from view to anyone who might come looking for me. I remembered Don's warning that so often wounded my ego: "You won't be able to walk out!"

"Oh God," I thought, "I could die out here!"

Veterans of the mountains had told stories about snowstorms, but I was a city slicker and had not taken their talk seriously. Now I wished I had paid more attention. As the car slid back, I grasped the steering wheel and put my foot on the gas, but it was too much and my rear wheels went into a skid. Whoa! Scary! I righted the car and eased off on the gas. There was a delicate balance of acceleration to keep me going forward without skidding out. I saw there was only one thing I could do. I just had to keep climbing.

Just as I was getting the feel for the gas pedal, the windshield wipers began to jam and snow was rapidly filling in the small peephole close to the dashboard. Soon that would close and I would be driving blind. "Jesus, Jesus, help me Jesus!" I stopped the wipers and started them, stopped them and started them, trying to get some clear window. I even rolled the window down and stuck the long-handled snowbrush out to knock some snow off the far left side of the window. Snow avalanched from the top of the car, and more came blowing into my face. I quickly rolled the window shut with one hand, still steering and delicately playing the gas pedal with my good right foot.

Now I was crouched over the steering wheel and staring intensely out the window as the adrenalin started to pump and my heart rate zoomed. I revved the defroster, trying to heat the window and melt the snow. "If I can just get to the ranch!" I thought. "Jesus! Help me Jesus!" The ranch was a wide spot in the road halfway up the mountain with an unoccupied house and a small field next to it. After the ranch, the road took another steep ascent. "Jesus, help me!" Under my coat, sweat was soaking my shirt.

Through my small patch of window, I saw a black shape emerge from the forest and step out onto the road. I gripped the steering wheel as the headlights flashed across it and gleaming eyes reflected back toward me. It was an elk with a huge rack, out for a stroll in the evening snow. Startled, he halted in the middle of the road, looking directly at me, surprised by the lights. At another time I might have admired this wild, magnificent beast, but now I was horrified by the imminent danger of colliding with him. I couldn't take my foot off the gas. I held my breath and just kept moving. "Get out of the road!" I shouted, earnestly praying he would move. He suddenly gathered his strength, tossed his antlered head and leapt across the road and down into the darkness. "Thank you Jesus!"

Another long, slow turn, then another surprise—headlights coming down the mountain! I was in the center of the road. That car might not be able to stop. I had to get out of the center. I gradually steered toward the right but didn't know how close I was to the ditch or whether there was enough room for the other vehicle to pass. Perhaps they would stop and help me. I rolled my window and waved my arm, but no, the headlights came quickly toward me, and as the truck pulled even I heard the sound of chains on the tires. They were prepared and I was not. They kept moving, apparently interpreting my distress signal as a friendly wave of the hand. As the taillights disappeared down the mountain, I felt even more alone. Why was I so stubborn? Why didn't I listen to Don? "Jesus, help me! Jesus! No! Don't slide back! Keep your eyes on the road. Keep on climbing!"

That night I learned respect for the mountains. I learned that you don't play around with danger. When you start climbing, you'd better have the guts to keep on going or you just might fall right off into space and never be found. I learned that I have inner resources to face a life and death struggle, but I also have limitations. I learned that when I use up everything I have, I need to look for a place, any place I can find, and pull over there and pray for rescue. That's what I did. I made it to the ranch, and I sat there exhausted and waited. Gradually my heart stopped pounding, and I took long, slow breaths, saying, "Yes, thank you, it's going to be okay now."

Sure enough, Don was in a turkey stew of worry on top of the mountain. He had been making phone calls to get some help. Before long, I saw the headlights of a pickup truck headed my way. It pulled up next to me, and out stepped John Davis, the site engineer, in his Western boots and wide-brimmed white cowboy hat, wearing a big grin. "Say, Lady, would you like a lift up the mountain?"

I AM Faith

Living in Sunspot offered plenty of object lessons for life. In contrast to the city, where contemplation occurred in the context of screeching traffic and fire sirens, the wilderness invited meditation on the natural things of life, sometimes by virtue of its beauty and sometimes by consequence of its tooth and claw rawness. After my experience on the mountain, I looked back at my life and thought that having MS is kind of like climbing a mountain in a snowstorm. You start climbing and you never know what will happen next. I wondered what it was that had got me through this far. I had come through a period of grief and despair and was now feeling better, both physically and emotionally. My meditations had brought me some peace of mind, and I wanted my improvement to continue. I didn't want to slide back down the mountain and over the edge into the darkness. I wanted the experiences and insights I had gained to have lasting value. I wanted to keep on climbing, but I could see that might not be an easy process—and that sometimes it might be downright scary.

An irksome question bothered me: Would the experiences and personal revelations that had begun to strengthen me carry me through future traumas of unknown nature and at unexpected times? With a disease like multiple sclerosis, the unthinkable could happen at any time. Or were my insights only temporary, theoretical snowflakes that looked pretty but would blow away in a blizzard.

I looked back through my notes and diaries to see what had triggered each of the positive changes in me. I saw that each stage of my growth and healing was accompanied by a remarkable experience of faith, almost a leap from doubt to assurance. I examined these experiences carefully. Some key phrases from my diary began to pop out at me that raised a lot of questions in my mind and helped me learn a great deal about the experiences of faith on my personal journey.

"I can boldly enter and remain in God's presence because Jesus is like me and fully understands me, even with all my handicaps."

"I just have to surrender to what God has already done. I have to agree with God. I have to say yes—in spite of everything."

"Like Jesus and Paul I must say yes to the present circumstances of my life, whether it is hard or easy or makes little or no sense."

"I must acknowledge my integrity… even if I am not my dream girl."

"I must open my eyes… even though before I open them I may expect to see nothing."

"I must allow the spark of life God has placed in me to grow and become strong and healthy, no matter how small and miserable that spark may look *at first in the great surrounding darkness."*

"I must have faith… even though I do not know what will come forth."

"I will be consenting to live life as the person I am now, even with all the complications and challenges that implies."

"I decided to say yes, not knowing what would follow."

One remarkable thing I noticed about these experiences of faith was that they seemed, at least to my first impression, to arise unexpectedly and at unpredictable times. Where did this faith come from? Was it the product of my own will, my own perseverance? Was it the power of positive thinking? What mechanism had allowed me to dredge it up out of the depths of my despair?

It did not take me long to recall the many times I had looked at the "Picture on the Way," the mental image I used over and over to try to imagine Christ and my relationship to him. Over time in that picture I had changed from a dogged, blind follower, to a friend, to actually being in the Presence of the I AM. I had been "looking" to the I AM from some different perspective at each of the crucial points when faith and growth occurred. Even in my blackest moments, to the extent I was able, and for as long as I was able, I looked to I AM. It seemed that the process of looking itself must have been faith, at least the primordial fetus of faith. Perhaps it was in me just because of the fact that I am a human being, created by God. I have a spark of God's being in me that calls me to look to the One who is the fullness of being and to believe that I can go on being.

In retrospect it seemed that looking to I AM is the only thing that produced any real faith, growth, or healing. The faith I tried to produce in myself by acts of will and by intellectual perseverance proved fruitless—in fact they were counterproductive. In previous times of my life a good positive attitude and physical perseverance no doubt helped me over many humps. But in the face of MS, such acts of will seemed to make me more sick and defeated. I could not control and focus my will strongly enough to accomplish things I needed and wanted to do. I could not conjure up enough faith to make God perform a miracle on me from the outside. I could not intellectually convince myself on the basis of available information that everything would be all right. Only looking to I AM produced real faith and, eventually, the real, deep-down healing of my whole personality.

So what was there about looking to I AM that was so powerful? I thought of all the "techniques" I had used, all the spiritual tools I had developed—dreams, meditation, research, memorization, introspection, dialogue, worship—and I realized that all of them were of no value in themselves. The real key was that I had set aside time to just be in the I AM Presence each day and that I had looked to I AM with all the strength and fullness of heart I had, even if it seemed to be little or none, and even if it did not seem very long or very effective. I had sensed the futility of hiding my real feelings, knowing I was completely transparent and that I might as well be honest. This meant opening myself to I AM in a radical way, confessing the truth of my being—both the good and the bad—and finding that I was fully loved and accepted. Faith came from being in the Presence.

As I continued my exploration of faith, I observed that certain phrases occurred frequently in my descriptions of the times when faith occurred. In the quotes above I noticed words such as "even though," "whether or not," "no matter how," and "in spite of." What did these "in spite of" phrases mean? Apparently they meant that I was saying "Yes" in the face of the obvious, imperious "Nos" that were confronting me. With the cool head of retrospect, I wondered if these were not the sorts of words that might eventually flee before the enemy, whether they might leave me sliding back down the mountain in a snowstorm. Where was their substance? Where was their content? Where was their intellectual foundation? They were quite unscientific, really—not to mention naive. They were words that flew their flag in the face of facts. If I were to say, "I'm going in the river, in spite of the fact that it's full of hungry alligators," or "I'm going to fly in spite of gravity," these would be foolish statements. I had in fact said, "I'm going to live, in spite of the fact that I seem to be dying." Is there a difference between the alligator and gravity statements and my decision to live? Was the faith that had produced these changes in me only fragmentary and temporary? Could I count on it to sustain me in the future? What if I found myself in an impenetrable darkness into which no ray of light could penetrate? What if I came up against a set of circumstances I could not leap over with the phrase "in spite of?"

I dug deeper. I asked myself what caused me to say yes in spite of everything to the contrary at each of the crucial turning points. Did I receive some promise of fullness of life, of healing, happiness, fame, or fortune to entice me toward the leap of faith? No. It was part of my frustration all along the way that I did not have any such promise. Was my yes at each juncture a wild step into the darkness based on nothing but wishful thinking and groundless hope? Was it just plain foolishness?

I decided it was not. At every crucial point God had stubbornly and uncompromisingly offered me the only thing of any value and efficacy—unconditional, irrevocable love. That love was manifested for me in the most profound sign I could imagine: Christ came to the earth and was born as a human being like myself so that he could know and understand my every need. Christ did this knowing that I could offer him nothing in return except my sin, my weakness, my disabilities. Christ accepted me and loved me in spite of myself, saying yes to me in spite of all my imperfections. I saw that my statements that I would live in spite of everything were based on the character of God, on God's unconditional love for me, not on anything God would subsequently do for me—or on anything I had done or would do for God.

Realizing that faith rises from unconditional love is like stepping from a deep forest to the edge of an infinite vista—freeing, empowering. I explored that vista with awe. As a disabled person I had been frustrated in how to express my faith in God because I was no longer able to express it in all the actions that are customarily associated with faith. I had made a terrible blunder: *I had confused the expressions or evidences of faith for faith itself.* When my physical disabilities disallowed all the valid expressions of faith that I knew about through works and doing, I made the awful mistake of thinking I had no faith at all—or that the faith I did have was without value. This confusion produced the horrible frustration and doubt that resulted in the massive identity crisis associated with my illness. If I could not work and *do* to express my faith, did I have faith at all? Could I sustain my faith if I was unable to express it through traditional works and doing? Would anybody know I still had faith? How could I find satisfaction in my faith if I could not *do* anything to show it?

The old doing-being dilemma sent me searching anew through scripture. I found passages that clearly describe how faith is expressed in ways other than by doing, performing, accomplishing, achieving, producing, and attaining—all the goals for which I had strived so long. I discovered that faith can be expressed just as profoundly—and perhaps even more so—by growing into the character and being of God. "Therefore, now that we have been justified by faith, let us *continue at peace with God* through our Lord Jesus Christ (Romans 5)." Peace with God is a response of faith that occurs in our *being*. Continuing in a state of peace is a valid and powerful expression of faith. I had experienced that this comes through being in the I AM Presence.

I also found that rejoicing in suffering is an expression of faith. Little wonder I had paid small attention to that! If I go out to feed the hungry and clothe the naked, I am fulfilled in expressing my faith. If I rejoice in suffering, some could think I am shallow, unrealistic, or even crazy. Who is happy about suffering? And yet, in the midst of my own suffering I found myself rejoicing in the love of God, in the Presence of I AM. The rejoicing was not an activity I chose or an intellectual argument I won—it was the inevitable result of being in the Presence. If I continued in the Presence, I could continue to rejoice, no matter what my circumstances would be and no matter if I ever *did* another thing in my life.

Further exploration revealed that there are many expressions of faith that are rooted in being and character rather than in actions and accomplishments. All the "fruits of the Spirit," the divine attributes of human character, come from faith: love, joy, peace, patience, kindness, goodness, faithfulness, gentleness, self-control—and many more. All of these are signs of faith, signs that a person is becoming more and more like God, growing in the divine image. I realized that this is the root and ground of everything. If actions and accomplishments are ever to come forth, they must come from the foundation of I AM.

The answer to the dilemma of doing and being was beginning to dawn on me, even though it would take me many years and a lot more suffering to understand and put it into practice. Faith is not doing *or* being, or doing *and* being. Faith is *becoming*, becoming one in character and Spirit with I AM. Faith means I keep on becoming All I AM.

Window Watcher

It was a sparkling, sunny day on the ski slopes, just crispy enough to keep the snow powdery, with a brilliant blue sky overhead. The slopes were dotted with the brightly-colored jackets of dozens of kids trying out their form, some wobbling in fits and starts down the beginner's hill to the left, some schussing down the intermediate path toward the right, and a few others hot-dogging like pros through the moguls that were just in sight up the center of the mountain. All the York men were on the bunny slope, just outside the lodge, getting their first ski instruction.

Ski Cloudcroft was a small resort east of the village where our kids were in school. It was a rudimentary arrangement in comparison with the big pro slopes farther north, but it was great for beginners. At 8500 feet, there was no guarantee of snow that far south in New Mexico, and the management had trouble keeping it open when it was a warm winter. In order to make a little extra money on off days, they arranged with the school to offer a Thursday special. Anyone in the school could rent basic equipment for five dollars and ski all day. The ski company could make money on ski lessons, food and upgraded equipment rental (the basic equipment was a little too basic for most people). Many kids in the district were poor, so the arrangement allowed the school to offer students a great experience that they otherwise couldn't afford. When the snow was on, everyone, including teachers, left the classrooms and headed for the slopes.

It was a holiday atmosphere. Out on the bunny hill it was melee and mayhem with all the greenhorn Yorks trying to learn the elementary ski moves. Don was out there with the boys, taking a day off to enjoy the kids' first ski experience. He had never been on a pair of skis in his life, so the whole gang was starting from scratch. Jeremy was the first one out, as usual, and he had already taken his first plunge down the hill and was extricating himself from the bushes at the bottom. Maurice was sitting on the snow between his skis, trying to get his boots locked in. When he got one in, the other ski went scooting down the hill. Being one who likes to think things through before taking action, he raised his eyebrows, looked at one ski and then the other, twisted his mouth to one side, and then, without further ado, slid down the hill on his bottom to catch the other ski. Oops! How would he get back up the hill again?!

Ski poles were a mystery to Chandler. After several attempts, he finally achieved an erect posture at the top of the bunny slope. He stood there gripping his poles, his legs a little too straight and stiff. Then, just a little weight shift, and whoops!—his legs slid wildly forward, ski poles flying in all directions. It was a three-point landing followed by a skid and a 180-degree sprawling rotation. Spectacular! Don, at 235 pounds, was the biggest bunny on the bunny hill. He was plowing toward Chan in slo-mo, laughing and calling, "Way to go, Chan! Show me how to do that!"—when his left foot slid out and he followed suit in his own inimitable style, letting out a whoop and landing next to Chan. They both sat there on the hill laughing, trying to help each other up, falling down again, laughing, showing each other how to do it, falling again, making a merry circus out of the whole escapade.

Meanwhile, Jeremy was getting the hang of it. With just a little instruction, he began looking like he was born to ski, bringing himself to a stop and doing modestly graceful turns in either direction. Before long he was headed for the rope pull on the beginner's slope. The older brothers saw him go, and, with renewed determination not to be outdone by the little guy, they soon mastered enough basics to get on the rope too. Don continued his exploits on the bunny hill and then happily headed for the rope himself.

It was a joyous occasion. I laughed at each spill and delighted in each little triumph. "What a crew!" I thought. "How lucky I am!" As the boys went off to try their new skills, they disappeared from my view, and I shifted my position, trying to catch sight of them through the big glass windows in the lodge. Then I was suddenly aware of my own situation. I was seated in a molded orange chair at a little square table that was littered with French fries and smudged with ketchup. My cheek and the palms of my hands were pressed up against the windowpane as I tried to get a view around the corner to where my guys had gone. My cane and scooter were nearby, but I knew the deck was too slippery for me to go out for a wider view. It seemed the joy was all happening out there on the mountain, all the color, all the sunlight, all the laughter. I was on the inside, looking out. The windows suddenly seemed small now that they no longer framed the ones I loved. I drew my cheek away from the window and let my hands fall in my lap. I was a window watcher, looking at an empty picture.

I AM Joy

Being a window watcher brought up a poignant question: "Will there ever be joy again, joy the way I've always known it before?"

Before I became ill, I was a person of intense feelings, indulging myself in a range of emotions that soared and plummeted with circumstances around me. I remember intense empathy with other people's experiences, and I recall strong surges of joy as well as acute frustration and hurt. When I became seriously ill, the emotional peaks and valleys flattened out. Intense feelings of any kind were too much for my nervous system to bear. The surges I identified as joy seemed to desert me. In fact, when I rarely did experience intense emotions, including joy, the emotional bubble would float for a short time, then burst, leaving me physically exhausted and emotionally fragmented. I discovered that I felt best when the highs and lows were all plowed off to the level of a flat plain. I did not know that the ability to experience equanimity, no matter what the circumstances, was regarded as highly desirable by great mystics of the past. I had no acquaintance with them. For me, the flat plain of ordinariness, in contrast to the emotionally charged landscape of my past experience, just seemed boring, like the miles and miles of Kansas plains we had to endure while driving out West. It caused me to ask the perturbing question: "Will there ever be joy again?" My free time in Sunspot allowed me to probe the question.

I tried to recall joyful experiences from the past and identify them by type to see if there was anything in them that could resonate with my current circumstances. Could I rejoice again, even in my weak physical state? Could I find an outlet for joy that wouldn't deplete and exhaust me? What provision of joy does God make for people like me? How could my joy be full when my body was so unresponsive and my prospects so uncertain?

I reflected on my experiences of joy in the past, and I saw a pattern that was quite enlightening. A few examples:

The joy of victory over an opponent. I recalled the joy associated with winning basketball tournaments as I grew up in Indiana—a joy so wild we called it "Hoosier hysteria."

The joy of personal achievement. I recalled the time when my drama team won first place in the state drama contest.

Physical joy. I thought of relaxing, warm bubble baths, taking a dip in cool water in summer, feeling my muscles work in running and hiking, experiencing the joy of intimacy in marriage.

Joy in receiving a wonderful gift. Of all the lovely gifts I have received from my husband, I recalled most strongly the joy of receiving my engagement ring.

Joy in excellence. Great music, drama and art often caused a surge of joy to spring up from deep within my innermost being. I rejoiced in the art itself and also in the spirit that created it.

The joy of beauty. Spectacles of natural beauty especially moved me to joy. I thought of the exquisite panorama of the stars spread above the Tularosa Valley at Apache Point.

The joy of fellowship. The warmth of family love and fellowship, especially during festive holidays, called forth a joy too deep for words.

Vicarious joy. I have often experienced great joy at the good fortune of other people, especially if it involves an experience of spiritual growth or transformation. Recently I had experienced the joy of my family having a great day skiing on the mountain.

I saw that each type of joy was based on activities, people, places and events in my life. Each of these experiences of joy was transient because actions and events occupy a finite time and place. They come, and then, fleetingly, they are gone, leaving behind the ache of a memory, a longing for repetition, a sadness that the joy has passed and that life has returned to bland routine. As soon as possible, I must seek further joy and greater satisfaction. I perceived that as I was growing older I did not seek just one thrill after another—I wanted quality. Often the quality that produces the greatest joy was elusive and rare.

I was amazed at these findings because, as soon as I looked at them clearly and objectively, I realized why I had had a dearth of joy in my life since I became disabled. As a healthy, doing person I sought out the things and events that gave me physical, emotional and psychological joy, as well as ego satisfaction. This was quite normal. Most of the things that gave me joy were wholesome pursuits, at least as long as I did not over indulge them. However, once I was no longer able to expend energy to go and do, I discovered that these joys were largely out of my reach. I could not seek out the activities, events, people or places that gave me joy. I hadn't the energy or strength to attend symphonies or operas, go to beautiful places, or interact with people I enjoyed being with, not even my dear mother, father and sisters. Due to fiery sensations on the surface of my body, physical pleasures that were once pleasant, even tender hugs or holding soft, cuddly babies, could now result in discomfort or pain. Physical movement was no longer satisfying but painful. I had to stop doing even some very sedentary activities, such as playing the guitar and crocheting, because my fingers were too sensitive and weak. Personal accomplishments were drastically limited or greatly changed. I had no sense of personal or communal triumph over obstacles and little opportunity to experience the vicarious joy of other people in my church or even of my own children in their various academic and athletic enterprises. As a result, I had little ego satisfaction. No wonder I saw life as being flat.

It seemed that only two circumstances might change this situation: I must either be healed so I could have the strength and energy to experience joy, or I must discover a joy that is independent of physical and time-locked events, actions and people in my life. It did not seem that physical healing was in the immediate future for me. What joy then could I find that transcends time and events?

I have often had the humiliating experience of looking all over the house for a pencil and then discovering one stuck behind my ear. A similar thing happened to me as I was looking for joy. One day I looked back over my notes and realized that I already had joy and that it was quite as accessible and functional as the pencil behind my ear. I had just failed to notice it was there.

How is it possible to miss joy? What I missed was the emotional exultation, the zip, the thrill, the buzz, the high. When my emotions were quiet, I made the terrible mistake of thinking joy was gone. It was true that I had been peaceful and content for months and that I was experiencing the love of God and God's care for me. It was true that I was happy with myself and everyone around me and that I felt I had come to terms with my disabilities, at least to a great extent. But I did not identify any of these as joy. They were not the thing itself. I knew quite well that all these circumstances could change overnight and that I could place no confidence in them. If my joy were in these, then joy is fleeting, momentary joy, and this was not the kind of joy I needed.

As I examined myself, I realized I was experiencing a long-term, bubbling-up joy, not a geyser that spouts off every now and then until it is exhausted, but a continual, clear, bubbling spring, washing through all my thoughts, days, relationships, and activities. I sought the source. It took me some time to realize that my joy was not coming from any external source or from any activity or accomplishment but from being centered and focused in my I AM Presence. The bubbling, continual joy I was experiencing was the joy that comes from the Spirit of I AM that is pervasive in me and everything I do or contact. I realized that previously I had measured whether God was with me by whether or not I could identify joy in the events and relationships in my life. In this sense, joy had been a kind of blip on a monitor measuring my spiritual health. As long as the blips kept blipping, I assumed I was okay. These blips were good reason to "do more for God." The more I did, the more fruit I could see, the more joy I could experience, the more objective evidence I would have that God was indeed with me.

My reflection revealed that for me as a disabled person this was a skewed perception of joy. The by-products of joy must not be confused with the Source of joy, the Personification, the Fullness of joy. This sort of mistake can lead to a type of service that is motivated by the search for emotional and psychological satisfaction, a geyser sort of experience—or, much worse, an ego sort of experience. As I found out the hard way, living for emotional highs and ego satisfaction was not a healthy lifestyle for me. Just after the mountain peak there was too often a fall off a cliff. It was also deceptive. When I am not experiencing emotional joy or the satisfaction of achievement, is God not with me?

I wondered how God's joy works, how it helps me live through everything I have to face. I realized that when I moved the question up into my head for analysis or out into my emotions to experience certain feelings, I was off center. It wasn't about blips on a joy meter. It wasn't about being a window watcher or a participant. God was working in a much deeper place than my emotions, intellect, actions and ego. God was working to transform me deep in my innermost being, in the place of my essence, my spirit, my being. Once again I was finding that the key to living a fulfilled life was in being focused and centered in I AM. The more I am centered, the more the life of I AM can infuse me, calm my thoughts, emotions and ego, and allow me to detect the subtle bubbling Joy deep in my innermost being. As that Joy bubbles up, it gives me strength to live, to will, to do, to be, to become.

Never Christmas

I reached up on the closet shelf and pulled down the one box we brought from Chicago labeled "Christmas." I told Don to bring only the favorite things because it was too much to ship back and forth. I carried the precious box into the little living room in our cottage and opened it on the brown couch next to the window. Outside there was a postcard Christmas scene, with snow piled in mounds on the roofs of the houses, icicles dripping in front of the windows, and tall pines with branches hanging low under the weight of snow. I could hardly believe it, but even as I glanced out the window, the picture was completed with a doe and two yearlings, sauntering across the road just a few steps from my door. I paused to enjoy the peaceful scene, so different from the bustling State Street at Christmastime in Chicago.

The men had gone on a Christmas tree expedition. There in the national forest you could get a permit to cut your own tree within certain marked boundaries. It was a way to allow people to cut trees and still maintain control over the place and number that could be culled. It wasn't easy work. All the good trees close to the road were gone, so getting a good one required hiking in, sawing and chopping it down, and carrying it back to the car. Good adventure for a troupe like ours.

I turned away from the window and looked inside the box. On top were the Christmas stockings, a big red one with a white fuzzy top for each boy, trimmed with gold braid inscribing his initials. I smiled as I remembered making them, creating a new stocking with the birth of each child. They were shaped differently because I learned as I went along that I needed a wider top in order to stuff the presents inside. I ran my fingers over the soft velvet and traced the gold braid. I had stopped sewing a few years before because my fingers were too sensitive to handle the fabrics. The stockings were beloved mementos of Christmases past. I laid them aside.

Next in the box were stuffed fabric tree ornaments that carried special memories. I had helped the boys cut them out and push the stuffing in, then sew up the hole and attach a string. I used to do a lot of crafts at Christmastime. As I touched each ornament, I recalled the happy times associated with it, and more memories came flooding in. I remembered the big gingerbread house we made one year that took up the whole center of the dining room table. All the boys and some of their friends got involved, stirring, cutting, baking, sticking the sides of the house together. I chuckled as I remembered trying to get the roof to stay on with pink and white icing. Red and green gumdrops dotted the roof, and little silver balls decorated the windows. One of the best things about it was the delicious smell of the gingerbread, filling the house throughout the Christmas season. When I closed my eyes, I could almost smell gingerbread. Then I thought, "Well, that's a thing of the past. I don't do those kinds of things any more." I didn't have the energy to manage them from my scooter. I smiled wistfully and thought to myself, "Those were the days."

My favorite thing of all was the Advent banner. I made it the Christmas after Jeremy was born and remembered doing the cutting and sewing next to the library fireplace in the Tudor house in Princeton. The blue felt background was bordered with blue and gold trim, and there

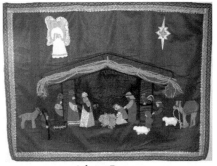

Advent Banner

was an outline of a stable in the center with gold yarn forming the straw of the roof. There were twenty-five handcrafted felt ornaments that could be velcroed to the banner, one for each day of Advent. Each day one of the boys got his turn to select an ornament and put it in place until the whole nativity scene was complete on Christmas day. There were shepherds, camels, white fuzzy sheep, wise men with removable crowns and gifts, a brightly plumed rooster to sit on the wall, and, of course, the Holy Family. The baby Jesus was always put into the manger on Christmas day. I unfolded the banner and hung it on the living room wall in our little cottage, placing a little tray of the ornaments next to it. Even in this far distant place, we would have a taste of home and tradition.

As I smoothed out wrinkles in the banner, involuntary tears welled up in my eyes. Yes, there was a postcard Christmas scene outside my window, and yes, my family was off on a big Christmas tree adventure. But I knew why I had told Don to bring only one box. I had learned over the years of being disabled that Christmas could be a heartbreaking time for me. I wanted to do so much to make it a happy occasion, but, because of my low energy, I always fell short of my own expectations. Bringing one box was my way of protecting myself so that I would not hope for too much and be disappointed. Bringing one box meant that I knew there would always be winter but never Christmas like it had been before.

I AM Hope

Hope is one of the last things I hoped for.

I have described how my illness gradually overwhelmed me, stealing from me my future, my past, and my present life. I have described that it was necessary to learn how to live one day at a time, never looking at the future, focusing my attention during each day on the practice of patience, endurance, rest, and peace for that particular day. During my Sunspot reflections, a paradox rose in my mind that I was unable to resolve for many months. If I am to be patient, enduring, restful, and peaceful, and if I am to live one day at a time, am I allowed to hope? If so, for what can I hope?

At the heart of my confusion was the fact that much of my hoping prior to this time was connected to the doings in my life. For example, I hoped I would be able to keep spending within our budget; I hoped we would be able to go to Indiana for Christmas; I hoped we would go to California on sabbatical; I hoped we would raise beautiful children; I hoped I could do certain services for others; I hoped I could teach a class well; I hoped I would have an easy, quick childbirth; I hoped for all the things young, healthy people usually hope for as they raise a family.

I also had a strong vision of what the world should be like. I hoped for a world in which there was justice and equality for all people, food for the hungry, healing for the sick, mercy for the downtrodden, and freedom for those in bondage. It was my hope that I would participate in bringing this to reality. I can't recall that any of my hopes were bad. Some of them were idealistic, even exalted.

When my doings were severely curtailed by illness, there seemed a vacuum of hope. Secular wisdom has it that at some point you must accept your condition in order to deal with it realistically and constructively. I believed God wanted me to do that. I was being pressed to cope with the status quo and, more than cope, to rest in it and find God's grace in it. I asked myself what hope is possible within those parameters? For example, I had taken to heart the scripture that says, "My grace is sufficient; my strength is made perfect in weakness." If this were true, I really wondered if I could hope for healing. If I believed I was to follow the Apostle Paul's example of being content in whatever circumstances I found myself, was I allowed to hope or plan for any changes? How far and how much could I hope?

While these may seem silly questions to healthy people, they were questions of psychological survival to me. If I hoped too much, and none of my hopes were ever realized, I might face horrible disappointment and depression. All my old hoping patterns were not working for me any more. They had been grounded largely in physical strength, in tangible, visible results. Now I was in a position of "helpless" hoping. Somehow the starch was taken out of my hope; it was a flimsy rag, blowing in a capricious wind. How could I learn to hope in productive, constructive ways? What did *God* want me to hope for? This is how I expressed my confusion to God in mid-November of 1988:

> *I wonder if I must always be satisfied with manna, never thinking of the finer table you have available. Am I to squelch the desires for a more varied, inspiring palate? Am I to deny that I know you have so much more available so that I can be thankful for what is in front of me? Am I to confess as sin my recognition of the goodness and richness of your gifts, and must I repent of my true belief that in your goodness, mercy, and forgiveness you would not withhold them? Am I remiss, having experienced peace, to desire joy, overflowing joy? Having found rest in your presence, should I not also desire inspiration? Having found patience, should I not also desire courage? And having experienced longsuffering, may I not yet aspire to service? Must my eyes always be turned inward and downward instead of outward and upward? Does patience and acceptance mean stagnation—or even just maintenance of the status quo? Having been exercised in trust, must I surrender hope? Having learned to be sustained, must I relinquish growth? I admit that*

wrongly motivated hope can skew destiny and neutralize the benefit of vision. But hope is one of the three enduring gifts. How can I employ hope judiciously as a partner with peace and patience?

I probed for answers to these questions. I found that my crippling illness had also crippled my hope. It was not that I had no hope; but I strongly disciplined it, corralled it, and spanked it into submission to the more necessary pursuits of survival. I didn't allow myself to hope for things that might disappoint me or to hope I would do things I might not be able to do when the time came. I didn't allow myself to dream very much.

I wondered what hope I could have that would not fail me. What hope could I have that would serve as the basis for joy and anticipation in all of life? I searched for an answer in a systematic way. In this case that meant I went into one of my paper-flinging, book-stacking, pen-scratching frenzies, studying all Old and New Testament scriptures about hope, outlining the meaning of the various Hebrew and Greek words used for hope, making lists of what I could and couldn't or should and shouldn't hope for. I stared at all the "chicken tracks" in front of me for several days.

Finally, it began to get through to me that Biblical hope is not the hope to have things or to do things. In the English language when we want or desire things or events, we can say we hope for them, and there is little difference in meaning. However, in the Bible, in both Hebrew and Greek, different words are used for desires or wants than for hope. Desires are directed largely to acquisition of objects or good conditions and toward the accomplishment of deeds or events. Desires often result in action, in *doing*, in order to bring the desire to fulfillment. On the negative end of the desire spectrum, the word "lust" represents evil or uncontrollable desire that often results in sin or usurpation.

Hope, on the other hand, seems to indicate an internal condition of the heart, an inward attitude, almost a view of life. Hope, in contrast to desire, is more a way of *being*. In the Old Testament, words translated as "hope" often imply waiting, patience and endurance rather than action toward a goal. Frequently, God is described as being the hope of a person or of the nation of Israel. The New Testament hope is Christ.

The distinction between desire and hope gave me considerable pause. I realized that my life as a healthy person was dominated primarily by desires, not hope. My desires served as a motivator to all kinds of doings, both secular and religious. When I became disabled, however, these desires were disappointing as prime motivators in my life; indeed, they constituted the root of most of my frustration and anger, because I could no longer accomplish or even attempt to fulfill them. On the other hand, hope, as it is referred to in scripture was an insipid little wraith in my previous life. When desires fell through the upper stories of the structure of my life, there was little foundation of hope upon which to rebuild. That seemed part of the reason why I was in a shambles for such a long time.

I could now understand why hope, along with faith and love, is one of the three most lasting and valuable of God's gifts, whereas desire is usually a product of the outer life and can give rise to all kinds of sin and unhappiness. Desire is based on material things and events that are elusive and disappointing in this life and of no consequence eternally; hope is based on things eternal, on the person of God through Christ and the Holy Spirit. If I live a life that is driven by desires, particularly as a handicapped person, I may be doomed to failure and despair. Hope, I concluded, is a good way to live, a good way to be.

Unfortunately, I didn't know how to start being hopeful. I didn't know how to live a life based on hope rather than desire. I reached deep into my past and my heritage and recalled the Spirit of Rising that had infused my early years. My heritage of resurrection hope, of going to heaven when I die, of being raptured out of suffering, all came back to me, and I explored whether this was the kind of hope I needed to re-kindle in my own life. The go-to-heaven-when-we-die hope was so deeply rooted in me and my religious genes that I had never examined it as an adult, especially from the perspective of a severely disabled person.

I spilled a lot of ink trying to work out my thoughts and feelings. When I looked back at my notes a decade later, I saw that I wrote more on that subject than on most others because it was so deeply ingrained in me. Initially I was very focused on the benefits of believing in the hope of resurrection to eternal life. I explored how it could help me as a disabled person live a good and righteous life right now because I knew I would be rewarded later. I explored the way it could deliver me from fear of death by knowing that there is something beautiful beyond the grave. I explored how it could comfort me in suffering by assuring me that suffering would end. I explored how it could help me delay the answers to my questions of "Why me?" by knowing that "We'll understand it all by and by." I explored how it would help me not to feel alone in suffering because the resurrected Christ suffered in the same way and is able to understand my pain.

All of that was a reiteration of things I already knew about hope of Resurrection, and the reiteration was good, as far as it went. It did give me comfort to meditate on these things. But many meditations later I came to the conclusion that comfort is one thing and strength to face the future here on Earth is another. The fact was that the well-ingrained hope of going to heaven that had been a part of my life since I was a child had not so far been very effective in helping me deal with terrible pain and despair in this life, here and now. When it came to my own suffering I wasn't content with resignation to my current circumstances while I waited for a reward after I die. I didn't want to shelve my possibilities in this life to wait for a future life when I felt there might be something I could still accomplish here. I wondered how streets of gold could help me get down my own street in a wheelchair or with a cane. I wondered how the promise that all tears will be wiped away in heaven helps me deal with my tears now. I wondered if it was necessary to lose myself in a world of heavenly dreams in order to escape the unpleasant realities of life on this Earth. So what if I have hope of heaven? What difference does it make to me in my quality of life, in the way I live right here on Earth now as a disabled person?

Finally, what helped me the most was when I realized that I had done to "hope" what I had done to my own life. I had focused on end goals and fulfilling achievements rather than on the One who had Resurrection power and who was able to give me that same power—not just in the future life, but right now. I was brought back again to that One who had been on the Way with me, that One who kept calling me back to the Center, back to the I AM.

The big thing that Christ did for me was to die and rise again, conquering Death, my most dreaded, mysterious, invincible foe. He had the Rising power. That power was most evident when he rose from the tomb on the third day, but the power of Rising was present before that. When he healed the sick, the lame, the blind, the lepers, and raised the dead, he was demonstrating that the power of Rising was available right then and there in the midst of everyday life and suffering. When he rebuked hypocrisy and meaningless traditions and demanded justice for the oppressed, it was Resurrection life powerfully breaking through into the politics and religion of his time. This is what Christ referred to as "the kingdom" or the "reign" of God. It was not far off in the distant future after this life was finished. It broke through whenever and wherever Christ was present. It was an environment in and around him. Whenever anyone entered that environment, it broke through in them too.

The power of Rising was manifest throughout Christ's trial and crucifixion as he pointed to a dimension of life far greater than that small stage on which his own painful drama was being played. The power of Resurrection Christ felt in himself is what moved him inexorably through the cross and through the grave, knowing and ever confident that there was victory on the other side. The triumph over the tomb was the ultimate expression of the power of Resurrection that had been operating in him throughout his life.

I asked myself the question: "If God's Rising power could break through in that world, why can't it break through in mine?" Christ said, "The kingdom is in you." If Christ is in me, the hope of Resurrection power should be a real possibility for me now. Why couldn't that Resurrection power work in me for whole, joyous, healthy, triumphant living in this life, just as it did for Christ?

It seemed to me that it came down to making a choice for Resurrection life. Christ was making that choice on the way to the cross and all the way through it. Even in the midst of struggle, pain and threatening, imminent death, he was affirming ultimate victory. I decided I needed to make that choice too. I wrote the following:

> *Resurrection hope energizes me to live as fully as I can now. We are not yet released from the necessities of the body in this world, nor from its pain or psychological traumas. However, when we feel peace in the midst of pain, joy in the midst of sorrow, or hope in the face of seemingly insurmountable trouble, we are experiencing the breaking through of the kingdom within us; we are holding within us a piece of eternity, of the life of God.*
>
> *Whenever we see a channel of mercy to the downtrodden, the hungry, poor, handicapped; whenever we see justice triumphing over prejudice; whenever we see freedom breaking bonds; whenever we see love lifting burdens and smashing barriers between races and nations of people, we see the kingdom of God breaking through. We see life triumphing over death.*
>
> *Whenever we are confronted with the choices of despair or hope in our physical struggles, and we choose hope, we are choosing Resurrection; we are saying yes to life and rejecting death. In making this choice, we are making the same choice Jesus made when he chose to go to the cross.*
>
> *When I as a handicapped person believe Resurrection has conquered death in all its forms, I am free to say yes to life in all its forms, to healing in all its forms. I am free to hope for the full gam-*

ut of life and all it can be, regardless of my own circumstances as they appear now. I can hope that God's bounty will break through on me and all of those around me. I can hope for divine intervention and healing in the midst of my patience and endurance. I can also hope that medicine and medical research will alleviate human suffering—even mine, especially mine. I can look for God's grace anywhere and everywhere, and in looking for it I can expect to see it in abundance!

I made a decision for Resurrection hope, and it was this decision that gave me courage and energy to live through the suffering of the next several years. I did not relinquish my hope of eternal life after death with Christ. Christ's assurance of Resurrection sustained him through the cross and through death. The Apostle Paul's hope of Resurrection kept him pressing on in the face of huge obstacles and eventual execution—and he did it with a physical disability. I decided I must press on too. But I decided to press on with the hope of Rising power here and now in this life as well. That is what life is all about. To stop pressing on would mean allowing my body to lapse into paralysis and living death. I decided I wanted the power of Rising to move me and fill me until it would be an environment around me and within me, overflowing in all parts of my life, energizing both my being and my doing and those around me, my hope for now and the future. I did not know what God would do with my life, but I did know that whatever I do—and whatever I am—I must be empowered by hope in the Presence of the Rising I AM.

Broken Neck

Sean came to Sunspot to share the Christmas season with us, bringing T-shirts, cups and other mementos of his first year at Northwestern University. I couldn't help being amazed every time I looked at him. My eyes were always searching him up and down, making sure he was really whole and strong after the traumatic injury that had nearly made him a quadriplegic during his senior year of high school.

I'll never forget the day when the phone rang and I picked it up to hear Don's voice at the other end, shaking and distraught. He was so upset that he didn't even attempt to cushion the blow for me. "Sean has a broken neck. They want to do surgery right away. They have him in a brace and won't let him move. Come to the hospital as soon as you can."

My heart began beating as though it would burst out of my chest, and a flood of adrenalin rushed through my body, initially making me feel somewhat woozy. I grabbed for the edge of my desk to steady myself and tried to take in what I had just heard. Horror gripped me as I suddenly envisioned a future for Sean in which he could be immobilized in a wheelchair, even more disabled than I. "No!" I shouted with every cell of my being. "This cannot happen! Please, God, don't let this happen to Sean!"

I pulled myself together and stood shakily to my feet. My MS symptoms were in a period of remission and I was able to walk short distances. I picked up my purse and headed out the door to drive myself to the hospital. When I arrived at Sean's room on the neurology floor, nurses met me with solemn looks as if to say, "Yes, we know it's touch and go, we're not sure what will happen now." I went in the room and saw Sean lying on the bed with a brace around his neck and Don standing on the other side of him, putting on a brave front for the sake of his son. I put on as good a smile as I could muster and moved to Sean's side. "Hey love, what's that thing on your neck?"

Sean's eyes rolled toward me. "They won't let me move my head," he said.

"That's okay," I said. "I'll move over here into better eye view. So what's going on?"

"Well, Mom, you remember last spring when that guy dropped me on my head at the party and I passed out?" Yes, I remembered. I recalled thinking it was a silly thing to happen and wondering what on earth what was going on at that party! We had called a doctor the next morning, and the doctor had asked, "Is he still able to move?"

"Odd question," I thought, but I answered in the affirmative.

On that basis the doctor concluded it was probably a muscle strain and recommended Advil. We didn't know until later that ninety percent of all people with Sean's type of injury are instantly paralyzed for life. The doctor felt that if Sean was still moving at all, there was little chance he had anything seriously wrong with him. We gave him Advil and he went on with his normal life and activities. As the summer progressed, however, he experienced more and more numbness in his right arm and side. In early fall he had an infection on the outside of his neck, and during treatment his pediatrician ordered an x-ray. When Dr. Samuels looked at the films, he couldn't believe what he saw. Sean's spinal chord was severely askew and resembled a dog's hind leg more than a human neck. He instantly called Don and told him to get Sean to the hospital immediately and to be very gentle in the process. Sean had been walking around for four months with a time-bomb neck that was ready explode him into a wheelchair for the rest of his life! Even a wrong step off a curb could have twisted the vertebrae just enough to paralyze him from the neck down. And he had been taking Advil for it!

As Sean and Don related the story to me, it seemed we were all perched unsteadily on a precipice, looking down into a dark, fathomless pit. One small misstep, one stone slipping beneath our feet could plunge us over the edge into a life of paralysis, lost dreams, lost hope. We held hands and prayed for God to hold us and draw us back to safety.

Now it was a year later and Sean was here before my eyes. Dr. Javad Hekmat-panah, (Dr. Hekmat to us) performed a cervical laminectomy on Sean and effectively stuck him back together so that he had nearly full range of motion in his neck and was all one functioning body. Yes, it had taken a long recovery, and we all had to work together to make it happen. It took such a toll on me that I went back into a wheelchair again, so that we had two invalids in the house at the same time, one of us wheeling slowly around, barely able to move, and the other stacking his plate on a pile of books in order to eat because he couldn't bend his neck. It was not an easy period of our lives. As a matter of fact, when Hannah Gray, the President of the University of Chicago heard about it, she felt it was such a tragedy that she gave our family a grant of several thousand dollars to help us get through the crisis. We used it to hire a part-time housekeeper who relieved the daily burdens of cooking and cleaning. We survived, all of us, and Sean had come through it all to live a normal life and attend college on time, like any other young man his age. When I looked at him, I saw a miracle.

I AM Love

Sean's ordeal caused me to reflect on my own experience of feeling separated from the human community that had been so important to me before my illness. I had felt the pain of being cut off from other people, alienated both from those in my church and from the larger body of humanity, like the phantom limb of an amputee. But Sean's experience gave me hope. By all accounts of the doctors, it was stunning and unexplainable that Sean had such an injury and was able to walk around with it for months without becoming a quadriplegic. Something held him together until he could get help, until someone with incredible expertise could glue him back together and make him back into one fully functional body, a whole person, able to actively participate in the world around him. I began to wonder, "If it could happen to him, could it happen to me?"

But there were no magicians for multiple sclerosis, no surgeons who could erase the lesions in my brain and spinal cord, and I had never heard of anyone being healed from this disease at an altar call. I couldn't imagine how I could be physically healed. But what about my social alienation? I wondered if one as separate from society as I could ever be a part of it again. I wondered if I, like Sean, could be stuck back together with the larger body of humanity.

I looked at a passage in the Bible that directly addressed my problem of body alienation, and I tried to understand what it meant for me. In this scripture (I Corinthians 12) the community of God is described through the metaphor of a human body. It says that the body is composed of many parts, such as eyes, ears, nose, hands and feet. It says no part of the body can be jealous of another and say it is going to switch over to being something else. For example, a hand can't decide it is no longer going to be a hand and opt to be a foot, because then the body would be without a vital part and could not function properly. Similarly, one part cannot say to another part, "Hey, I'm better than you! You're not needed any more!" Every part is necessary or the body will not work as intended. Even if a part is not as attractive as another, no one can deny that it is important. For example, the tongue is not a particularly beautiful part if you look at it by itself, but it is a big loss if one can no longer speak. The parts that seem to be less attractive and have less honor need to receive special care from the others so that there is no part that is cut off from the rest. The passage ends with the assurance that every person in the community has special gifts to offer and is a vital part of the body.

"Alright," I thought, "so I'm an essential part. I may not be so beautiful, but I am a part, and it doesn't do any good to wish I could be some other part. I am what I am. So what does that mean?" I thought about it. What did I have to contribute as a disabled person that was unique and could not be contributed by anyone else?

I recalled the way I had viewed disabled people when I was a "healthy-normal" person. I realized with shame that I had always thought of disabled people as offering a good opportunity for the rest of us to minister to them, to be the "hands of Christ" reaching out to them, exercising our gifts of kindness, compassion, gentleness, and humble service. We were the givers and they were the receivers. From where I was sitting now (in an electric scooter) I was offended by that self-centered, self-righteous attitude. I didn't like the idea of being the ladder on which other people could ascend to a higher state of spirituality and self sacrifice. I didn't want to just be a receiver—I wanted to also be a giver! But what did I have to give?

I looked down at my own body. Once again, I faced all the old doing and being dilemmas. My feet were no good, sometimes my hands were no good. I had little strength. I couldn't go and do and work and play and serve like other people. I sat there, turning my hands back and forth, looking at them, looking down at my feet, stroking my legs lightly with my fingertips, pursing my mouth, sighing, running my hands up and down my arms, thinking about these body parts and feeling frustrated that they were so weak and feeble. Hmm. I closed my eyes and got very quiet. As the stillness deepened and I let go of my thoughts and frustration, I became aware of my breathing, in and out, in and out, in and out. I took a deep breath and let it go. Then I began to feel my heart beating, ka-thump! ka-thump! ka-thump! until it seemed like it was pounding in my ears, KA-THUMP! KA-THUMP! KA-THUMP! When my stomach growled, it sounded like a roar in a canyon, reverberating around my body and out into the room, bouncing off the walls and rattling the windows.

My eyes popped open! I had been so focused on my outer body members—my hands, arms, feet, legs—that I had forgotten I have *inner* members as well—brain, heart, lungs, stomach, kidneys, liver, intestines. What about all of these parts! They are vital organs the body can't live without, but they are hidden on the inside, doing their work of nourishing, cleansing, balancing, and energizing out of the view of other people. As I thought about it, my old doing and being dilemma seemed to be taking on new dimensions. Now I could see it was not just about the outer, active, visible members of a body but also about the inner, hidden, vital parts that make it possible for the rest of the body to function. Certainly if any of the vital organs are missing or even damaged, the body is impaired in its function. Perhaps in the community of humanity I was one of the hidden but vital organs that was giving life to the whole in some way I had not even suspected all this time.

My meditation continued, extending not through a single hour or day but through many days and weeks. I became accustomed to using my physical body as a metaphor for thinking about my relationship to other people. I looked at it inside and out, upside and down and around and around. Eventually I began thinking about the parts of myself that are not only invisible to other people but also intangible—my mind, my spirit, my heart, my character. I noted that my mind is the faculty that thinks, reasons, analyzes, remembers, visualizes, imagines, and so much more. My spirit connects me to the spiritual dimension that includes my perception of God. My heart (or emotions) allows me to express feelings toward myself, other people and God. My character is the sum total of my personal qualities that I have built through every action, thought, choice and feeling I have ever had. I realized that these intangibles, these qualities that constitute my essence, make me unique from every other person who has ever lived. How then could these unique essentials connect me back into the human community and make me part of the whole?

One day I was looking once again at the passage in the Bible about the members of the body. My eye went on past the end of the chapter and started reading the next one, I Corinthians 13, the chapter on love, one of the most beautiful in all scripture. It was a scripture I knew by memory but, for some strange reason, had not connected with my own issues of being a disabled person in community:

> *"If I speak in the tongues of mortals and of angels, but do not have love, I am a noisy gong or a clanging cymbal. And if I have prophetic powers, and understand all mysteries and all knowledge, and if I have all faith, so as to remove mountains, but do not have love, I am nothing. If I give away all my possessions, and if I hand over my body to be burned, but do not have love, I gain nothing."*

This told me that my struggle to be connected lacked the single most important ingredient, without which nothing else mattered. I had been so focused on my own loss of physical function that I had moved the center of importance to outer manifestations and had failed to address the true center, the essence, the heart of all things, Love. "Yes," I thought, "God is Love."

I stopped to take in the meaning. I had the feeling that the Universe had been very hazy and ill defined for a very long time, and it was now coming into focus, as though the lens of a telescope were moving into place and suddenly the whole sky would be brilliant with planets, stars and galaxies. Love. That was the answer.

But what did it mean for me? I read on:

> *"Love is patient; love is kind; love is not envious or boastful or arrogant or rude. It does not insist on its own way; it is not irritable or resentful; it does not rejoice in wrongdoing, but rejoices in the truth. It bears all things, believes all things, hopes all things, endures all things."*

This was saying that love must infuse every aspect of my being. It didn't matter whether I was going or doing or being or thinking or feeling or having faith or good character or anything else—outer, inner, visible or invisible, tangible or intangible. If it was not full of love it meant nothing.

I struggled with the passage long and deeply. It would have been nice if I had just been able to say "Oh yes, love. Of course! I'll do that this afternoon." But of course it wasn't that easy. I discovered why I hadn't connected this particular passage with my own need for community. When I probed into myself, I saw that it was anger that was creating so much of the alienation I was experiencing. Ghoulish emotions were imprisoned in my heart, clawing at my insides, clamoring to be set free. All the times when I wanted to go and do and was locked up in a body that had betrayed me. All the times when I wanted to just be a normal person but drew only looks of pity. All the times when I wanted to join the fun but had to sit on the sidelines. All the times I wanted to create and contribute, to be a giver, but had to passively receive. All the times I knew there was something in me that could uplift others but no one could see past my crippled exterior. All the frustration, hurt, tears, pain, brokenness, defeat—they all worked their way up from the depths, seeking escape.

When the anger started to come out, it was like a bear out of hibernation, hungry and dangerous, looking for prey. I knew I didn't want to just fit back into things and be accepted like everyone else. No, no, that wouldn't be enough! I wanted to blame somebody, everybody—blame the world for all the pain and rejection I had experienced. I wanted to rebuke, reproach, reprove, reprehend, remonstrate, berate, vituperate and castigate until I exhausted the thesaurus. Even more, I knew that blaming wouldn't be enough. What I really wanted was payback. I wanted the satisfaction of others acknowledging how they had hurt me, ignored me, patronized me. I fantasized some groveling, some cowering, some people down on their knees in front of my scooter, their hands clasped, their eyes full of tears, their voices shaking and remorseful, their faces turned up to me, confessing their "sins of omission and commission" as they used to call them in prayers when I was growing up. I envisioned them declaring how wrong they had been, how insensitive and blind for not realizing what an amazing person I am. I wanted to hear them say, "Oh yes, we've hurt you so bad, we were so unjust, so evil, scum of the earth, pigs in the trough! We'll make up for it! We'll start building a handicapped ramp tomorrow! We'll give you your own parking space!" I wanted to personally hear them pleading for forgiveness at the mercy seat, and then begging me to please, please come back and bless them with all the abundance of my wonderful gifts. Then I wanted to graciously, humbly shed my benevolent forgiveness on them, receive them into my loving arms and take my rightful position at the center of the community. I wanted satisfaction! I wanted compensation!

So now it was out! Confronted with the purity of the demand for love, the beast inside me was rearing up on its hind legs, waving its paws and roaring at the wilderness. Deprived too long, the first thing I wanted to do was make noise. I roared it and then wrote it, filling page after page with descriptions of how it feels to be an outsider, to be alienated, to be a non-person. I wrote advice—volumes of advice!—about how people, especially churches, should strip the blinders from their eyes, repent of their indifference and self-centeredness, re-shape their ministries to empower the weak instead of satisfy their own egos, and reach out toward people like me as equals instead of underlings. Maybe they would see what it is like one day if they became disabled!

When the writing had sufficiently tamed the roaring and the wilderness was quiet once more, I leaned back on my haunches and licked my wounds. Eventually, as I calmed down, I came back around to that love chapter again, perhaps thinking I would see something there to justify my rage. Surely there must be an escape clause for injustice! But when the dust settled and the air cleared, I saw I had read it from a seriously flawed perspective. My anger had caused me to interpret it as being addressed to everyone else out there who hadn't treated me as I wanted to be treated. I was blaming everyone else for not loving and was conveniently removing myself from the target of the pointing finger. Now that my anger was expressed and my adrenal hormones were returning to normal levels, I humbled myself and saw all of the rest of my own fingers pointing back at me. I read all the way to the end of the chapter, and I allowed the words to speak directly to me: "When I was a child, I spoke like a child, I thought like a child, I reasoned like a child; when I became an adult, I put an end to childish ways." My roaring had been the cry of a hurt child inside me. Could I let go of the hurt and move on to a more mature, open, accepting, mutual relationship with the people around me? For a long time, I did not know.

Slowly, I came to grips with the fact that if that were to happen, if I were to be re-incorporated into my church and the larger human community, I couldn't passively wait for others to show me love first. I didn't see any "if-then" clauses in the love chapter. It was calling me to total, complete, now and forever, unconditional love, calling me to embody love in every part of myself, my goings, doings, feelings, thinkings, inner, outer, upper, downer, visible and invisible, tangible and intangible parts, no matter what other people might do. It was calling me to make love my hallmark, my watchword, my manifesto for living. Did I know how? No, I did not, but that was okay. I would find out as the future unfolded before me.

Rising and Falling

Up and Down the Mountain

Mountaintop experiences can be times of great insight and inspiration, but there is nearly always a harsh wake-up that follows when one comes back down the mountain to "real" life. There is a story of that sort associated with Christ's transfiguration. Peter, James and John were the three disciples who were closest to Christ. One day Christ took them with him into a high mountain and allowed them to see into the spiritual realm, viewing him transfigured in great radiance and talking with Elijah and Moses, two great spiritual prophets of the past. A voice spoke from heaven, telling them the import of what they were seeing. It was an overwhelming experience for them, one which they did not understand, but which certainly changed them and began to prepare them for the events that were to come in Christ's life and in their own lives.

The disciples' experience of transfiguration glory was short lived. They came down from the mountain wondering what happened to them, unable to internalize their experience. At the foot of the mountain they met with life's harshest realities in the form of an uncontrollably epileptic child. To their dismay, the experience on the mountain did not give them the power to heal the child. They were directly confronted with their own weakness and lack of faith. It would be some years before they understood the meaning of what happened on the mountain and how they were to put their spiritual power into action.

This story of going up and down the mountain provides a metaphor for my experience during the next few years of my life. The powerful inner life of the I AM that began to grow and flourish in my innermost being took me up the mountain, a place of insight and empowerment; the death that gradually began to take more and more control over my physical body confronted me at the foot of the mountain. I traversed that path, up and down the mountain, time after time, gradually gaining more insight, but always returning to the harsh realities of life with a progressing disability.

We came down the mountain from a year's sabbatical in New Mexico and experienced culture shock as we re-entered urban life in Chicago. It wasn't long before we were all caught up in the same hectic lifestyle we had before our departure—work, school activities, travel. While I was in Sunspot, my health had improved overall, even though I had broken my leg when I tripped on some magazines in the living room. I was healing well. Unfortunately, it was not long after I touched down in Chicago that I began deteriorating. My Sunspot reflections on Faith, Hope, Joy and Love gave me a *spiritual* manifesto for living, but my *physical* body was still a complete mystery to me. I had no idea how to nourish my body and guard my energy, so I was always overextending myself physically. I had the idea that if the Spirit were strong enough in me—if I went up the mountain for long enough—God would make my body strong. I did not understand that my spiritual energy needed to be in balance with my physical strength and that I needed to create and sustain that balance by implementing healthy lifestyle choices. Therefore, I pushed forward in expressing my spiritual energy but ignored the needs of my increasingly weak body.

I began to experience more frequent and more severe MS attacks, sometimes as many as six a year. I would have no time to recover from one before another would strike. My lower left side became increasingly weaker until my left hip and leg were largely paralyzed. The sensations in my feet were so fiery that I could not touch my feet to the floor without severe pain. I began to use my electric scooter regularly, even to get from the bed to the bathroom. My muscles atrophied until my legs began to resemble spindly sticks. My left leg became twisted from lack of use and from the constant seated posture. When I did walk, I used a cane and developed a serious rotation downward and to the right from my habit of leaning on the cane. I became very sensitive about my appearance and did not allow photos of me sitting in a scooter or wheelchair. In spite of the pain, I would always stand for long enough to have a picture taken. I attended a few meetings of MS support groups at the University of Chicago Hospitals, and I met some people there who were struggling valiantly with the disease. Most of them were long-time MS sufferers and, like myself, were in a state of continuing deterioration. I stopped attending because I couldn't get to the meetings without help.

My disease progressed until, by late 1994, I was so weak I could not even sit up straight for more than fifteen minutes. I did my work from a partially reclining position in a chair that rolled, revolved and reclined so I could have everything at my fingertips without getting out of the chair. Sometimes my hands and arms were so weak I had to wear braces on both the left and right hands. Most of the time I was able to type on my keyboard, but there was a period of time when even that was impossible. I lived daily with pain that was often excruciating, including shooting nerve pain and random electrical tingling that made me feel like I was plugged into an electrical socket. Flickering eyes caused fatigue during reading. The difficulty of performing each task required careful concentration, so I was unable to focus on more than one thing at a time. Noise, movement and stress in my environment distracted me from concentrating on what I was trying to do and made me feel frustrated and fatigued. I interspersed periods of work with periods of rest in order to accomplish any task.

Getting my own food together was challenging, because I had to prepare and cook it from a seated position. Getting it from the kitchen to the dining room on the scooter was a juggling act in which I feared all the pieces would go crashing to the floor at any moment. When I was eating, I often needed to lift a glass or plate with two hands, and I even used a lightweight fork and spoon.

I lost the ability to perspire, a condition which made me extremely sensitive to conditions of heat and cold. When I went out of the safety of air conditioning in the summer, I would carry a large cup of ice and would rub the ice on my face, arms and legs to cool down. Sometimes I carried a spray bottle with which I would spray myself all over, including my clothing, to create cooling moisture on my skin. In winter my limbs had a deathly chill. Once I became cold, it was hard to get warmed up, requiring a hot bath or an electric blanket. On the other hand, during periods of stress, I experienced surges of electrical heat that felt like it was frying the wires of my nervous system.

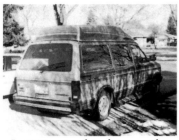

In 1995 we purchased a van with a wheelchair lift.

In March of 1995, we purchased a van with a wheelchair lift in the hope that I would be able to go places somewhat independently. In fact, that did not happen, because I could not get out of our building and into the van without help, especially when it was snowy outside.

I took several types of drugs, including tranquilizers and steroids, and some of them had side effects almost as bad as my disease. There were times when I had to go to the hospital for intravenous steroid treatments. It was during this time that I had MRI's that showed multiple lesions on my brain and spinal cord, the internal evidence of my neurological failure. This was life at the foot of the mountain.

In contrast, my spiritual life was flourishing. After Sunspot I began to express myself once again through poetry. These expressions had somewhat the character of Biblical Psalms in that they expressed both the depths of hurt and pain and the heights of praise, thanksgiving and faith. As I review these expressions, the life and death struggle in which I was engaged comes through profoundly. On the one hand, I expressed the horror of having a deadly, crippling disease that was completely out of my control. I expressed my desire for release from my painful body, but, practically in the same breath, I also called for renewal and healing.

> *There's a powerful death at work in me, compelling me to the grave;*
> *It began at birth and curses my life, and causes me pain and grief.*
> *I have no will nor fortitude this monster to restrain.*
> *It has its coils around my heart and its claws inside my brain.*
>
> *This mortal flesh groans in its fight to be clothed on with Christ,*

To shed this painful, darkened house and receive its robes of Light.
Who is able to deliver me from the body of this death?
O Spirit of God, come blow on me with your cleansing, hopeful breath.

I knew in my innermost being that God was guiding my destiny, and, even in the midst of suffering, I captured glimpses of possible transformation.

Transforming love, I can't explain the newness you impart,
Breaking in with life where my hope had died,
Refreshing me with living springs of joy,
Restoring me with healing oil.
Amazing God, I give my all to you.

Compelling love, how can I not surrender all to you,
When your Spirit flames in my trembling frame!
All I am and have, yes, all I hope to be,
O God who guides my destiny,
Compelling God, I give my all to you.

If I had graphed the relapsing-remitting progress of my disease during these years, it would have mapped as two lines, one for my spiritual life and one for my physical condition. Both would rise and fall as I went from weaker to stronger, from sickness to health, from hurt to hope and back, again and again and again. The overall direction of the spiritual line, however, would be rising, always rising, while the physical line was falling, falling, falling.

Coming Together

Shanta Premawardhana was a different sort of person than I had ever met in my life. An immigrant from Sri Lanka, he had become the pastor of our church while we were away for a year in New Mexico. Part of my new spiritual outlook included the hope of becoming more a part of a community, and my first meeting with Shanta heralded a new era of acceptance and participation. He was able to look through my exterior disabilities and see the person inside. He began to explore my gifts, especially those that focused on prayer, and began to empower me to use them. Shanta was to become the key figure in the development of my outward spiritual expressions and ministry for the next fourteen years, serving as my pastor, mentor and friend, and eventually opening the way for my ordination to ministry.

My ministry first began to flourish in our Wednesday evening prayer and Bible study time, which became focused more and more on prayer. Right there in that small group we had some of the most challenging, serious situations that either of us had ever dealt with—or expect to deal with in the future! We had persons struggling with severe alcoholism, drug addiction and drug pushing, multiple personalities, homelessness, domestic violence, rage, and ex-convict employment issues. My upbringing had schooled me to believe that God can do anything, and that belief seemed to be a magnet for people with problems. My heart reached out to serve beyond my physical capacity to deliver. I was fool enough to think that I had strength to be the vehicle for healing such serious situations when I myself was so physically fragile. I spent hours ministering to various individuals, usually in the context of my home, since I was not strong enough to go out. My inner strength, faith, patience, and perseverance began to manifest outwardly in the transformation of other people's lives. Unfortunately, I did not know how to protect my own energy so that I could sustain such intense ministry. I was spending my energy freely, thinking I was drawing on an infinite checking account, but I was drawing down my balance with too small deposits to keep me viable. The huge amount of energy required to minister to those in such tragic circumstances sent me into deficit spending, and I became physically weaker and weaker.

Besides those with severe problems, there were several individuals and couples in the church who were hungry for spiritual revival. In spite of my weakness, or perhaps because of it, the life of Christ in me shone brightly enough for other people to want the kind of hope and faith they saw in me. One Sunday afternoon a beautiful young mother came to me, expressing her need to know God in a more personal, intimate way. She said it this way: "Anna, I don't know what it is you've got, but whatever it is, I want it." Soon this woman's husband sought me out, and then others as well. These people, who were leaders in the church, became part of a cell group that met at our house. I mentored them in prayer, Bible study and the gifts of the spirit, and they began to experience powerful transformation in their lives and ministries. Old sins came to light and were cleared; seemingly impossible obstacles were overcome; and we experienced spiritual and emotional healing, as well as healing in relationships.

Along with the victories, creativity began to flow in our small group and in the larger context of our church. A new song was born in my own heart, and I shared it at a Wednesday night prayer meeting:

When you break through in me,
Through all my fears,
You open my possibilities
Into your sovereign freedom.
You're not impressed with my limitations,
And you decide what you can do with me.
When you break through in me,
O Lord, you set me free.

I was filled with a profound gratitude that the song in my heart was restored after so many years of spiritual dryness and physical duress.

When my spirit is dry and my heart is a stone,
And melodies die that sustained me so long,
I wonder through all the heartache and pain,
If I'll ever know how to praise You again.

When the branches are bare, and the fruit I have borne,
Is too bitter and small to share with a friend,
The breath of a prayer that rises within
Reminds me that God can restore me again.

Then the healing begins like the trembling of wings
Of a long-silent lark, remembering to sing.
I'm thankful for grace that breaks through my pain
And opens my eyes to Jesus again.

Chorus:
I'm singing again, after all I've been through,
Singing again, a new song to You,
Like flowers in early spring,
The Spirit's refreshing rain,
Has opened my heart to music.
The wilderness lives!
I'm singing a new song to Jesus, my king.

I shamelessly, joyously shared my musical creations, regardless of how unprofessional they were, and others began to capture the spirit of it, gaining hope and courage to bring forth their own creative expressions. Many people began creating original songs and sharing them, first in the group and then in the larger congregation. Those talented in music would set them to music and develop arrangements for guitar and other instruments. Eventually, a music ministry team came together and a worship style blossomed that was completely unique to our congregation. Even children wrote and sang their songs. Other gifts flourished as well. Peggy, an artist, began to create art for our bulletins and for sanctuary decoration.

Since I was not able to bear the burden of ministry alone, I tended to create teams to accomplish various tasks of service. Eventually we became a "teaming" church, drawing groups of people together to address serious situations so that no one person had to carry the load of ministry alone. These teams addressed a wide range of needs, some of which included homelessness, gang rape, partner violence, dysfunctional families, and even a victim of a lab explosion. I coordinated these teams by phone from my reclining office chair and was a member of most of them. Sometimes one of the people in crisis would stay in my home for a period of a few days to a few months. Even when I was the most ill, we had a constant flow of people through our home.

In the meantime, the small group that met in our home grew into a large group. In its heyday, before we broke into smaller groups, we had about twenty adults meeting in our home each week, plus babysitting service in one or more other locations. We called ourselves the "Mitochondria," a scientific term for the genetic material that is common to all human life. We ministered lovingly to each person's and each family's needs, and members of the group ministered tenderly to me and to our family. They brought us meals when I had to go to the hospital and helped with transportation and other needs. The church purchased a reclining chair so I could sit comfortably in the sanctuary during worship services.

Prayer ministry was powerful among us for whatever need arose. One night especially stands out in my memory. We had a white Flokati shag rug on our living room floor, and those in the small group would sit cross-legged on it for prayer, gathering in a close circle in which we could feel the tangible love that flowed among us. We shared the secrets of our souls and reached out to lay hands on one another, praying with loving tears for Christ's healing and wholeness in our lives. We had many answers to prayer and many healings, all of which increased our faith and love. On that particular night, I was facilitating the meeting from a big green Lazy Boy recliner, and after we prayed for various ones, I shared that I was having a new MS attack. Around the circle, every face expressed sadness and concern. Their shoulders sagged with the weight of the news. "Not again!" was the unexpressed exclamation. They sat there quietly for a moment, and I felt their hurt that I was once again moving into a time of increased pain and weakness. I wanted to say, "It's okay, dear friends, it's okay," but I wasn't sure it was. I just let them be present with me. Then Karen and John disappeared into the kitchen. After a moment, they reappeared, and with a tender smile Karen said, "Well, Anna, we're going to pray for you and anoint you with oil. So we want you to lie down on the floor."

I gave a gentle laugh. "Sure. Where do you want me?" I was usually the one who was calling for special prayer for other people. Now they were taking the lead for me.

"Right there in the middle will be fine." I released the handle of the recliner and slid down onto the Flokati, rolling over on my back. Someone put a pillow under my head and another under my knees. Then everyone gathered around, sitting cross-legged or on their knees. John had brought some olive oil from the kitchen in a small bowl. He said, "Anyone who wants can put their fingers in the oil and say a prayer while we anoint Anna."

The prayers started with soft, rhythmic phrases. "Thank you Jesus. Praise you Jesus. We bless your name, Lord. You're our healer, Lord. We praise and thank you. Hallelujah! You're right here Lord. We feel your presence. Hallelujah. Glory to your name. Thank you for loving us Lord. Pour out your Spirit Lord. We love you so much Lord. You give us everything you are. You don't hold back anything. You love us so much. We praise and thank you Lord."

The air in the midst of the circle became warm and vibrant with love. It seemed like there were no longer individuals praying but that the group had one heart, one soul, one will, seeking God's healing for one they loved. "Thank you Lord. Yes Lord." I surrendered myself into their loving embrace and into the bosom of the Spirit that seemed to cradle me so tenderly. John was the first to dip his finger in the oil and then gently make the sign of the cross on my forehead, all the while praising and thanking God. Then another reached in and anointed my temples. Another took my hand and, placing it in her own, began to rub oil into my palm and all around the fingers, then on my wrist and up my arm. Soon all formality and inhibition was gone. From around the circle hands reached into the oil. Both of my hands were bathed in oil. My head, my hair and neck were anointed. Someone gently removed my socks and began to massage my feet, praying they would receive strength, walk and leap. Then Karen said, "Anna, I want to anoint your back and spine." I turned over on my stomach, and, as they all closed their eyes, the group began to hum and then sing softly, "We love you, Lord, and we lift our voice, to worship you, O my soul rejoice. Take joy my King in what you hear. Let it be a sweet, sweet sound in your ear." Karen slipped her anointed hands under my shirt and began to massage my back, all down the sides and then down the center on my spine. It was just plain olive oil they were using, and the season was winter. Nevertheless, as the prayers ascended, the room was filled with the delicate scent of roses, as though a window had been opened on the gardens of heaven. The scent lingered in the air. The healing angels were pouring out their love. A deep quietness enveloped us, and I rested in the beauty of the moment as though it would never end, deeply touched by the power of love.

The prayers ended gently. Quietly and reverently, each person went home with a heart full of faith and hope. I rested in peace.

At that time I thought that life together in this group came as close as anything I had ever experienced to expressing true community. I wrote about it in a song that became somewhat of a theme song for our diverse church.

> *Look around and see how different we are,*
> *The color of our skin and hair, the accents of our speech.*
> *But in spite of all our differences, we're learning how to be*

One body, one spirit in love. (Chorus)

Here and now we see a mystery unfold,
The walls between us disappear as Christ is formed in us.
Our races, creeds, and genders yield to reconciling grace;
Forgiving, healing, we are joined in peace. (Chorus)

We're created in the image of our God,
Who dwells within our human flesh, becoming one with us.
When we can bridge our differences and join in unity,
We're imaging the glory of God. (Chorus)

Look around and see how similar we are!
The Spirit joins us heart to heart in laughter and in tears.
Our gifts unite to serve and praise the God whose life we share,
Who binds us in one body in love. (Chorus)

Chorus:
We're coming together in love,
Discovering God's purposes here and now,
Rejoicing in diversity and building community,
We're coming together in love.

Coming together in community healed the hurt I had experienced of feeling like an outsider because of my disabilities. It was the fulfillment of my hope that I, even I, a struggling person with a severe disability, could find loving fellowship—but more than fellowship—meaningful ministry that empowers others.

My physical healing did not happen on that magical evening of angels and roses, nor did it happen for a long time to come. Support from friends gave me inner courage and strength to continue my journey, but it was a path of physical pain and weakness.

Everybody's Mom

I heard a hubbub in the hallway, dropping boots, a key in the lock, and then the raised volume of voices as the boys and their friends poured through the door, harassing each other in the manner of teen males. "Man, what was Coach into with that swim-the-length-of-the-pool-underwater stuff!"

"I got half way and man, I thought I was going to explode all over that pool."

"You can't take it, man! You gotta be strong like me!"

"Yeah, yeah, right!"

All the chatter was quickly followed by, "Hi Mom!" Chandler came into the sunroom and gave me a hug, followed by Brent, a black swim team brother, the fastest guy on the team. Brent said, "Hi Mom" and spread his arms out to offer a hug right after Chandler. Behind him was Paul, greeting me with a big grin. "Hi Mom! How ya doin' today? Got any cookies?"

I sometimes wondered if I had the word "Mom" printed on my forehead. My husband, my children, all their friends, and everyone I knew at church and in the community called me "Mom." Even people I didn't know came up to me and called me "Mom." My soft body was a mom's body and my soft heart was a mom's heart. Everybody wanted to hug me, and when they did so, I would give them a big, warm, mom's hug in return.

Our house was "home" to a lot of people. We lived just a couple of blocks from the kids' school, so it was easy for them to come home for lunch or after school, bringing their friends along for snacks, studying or video games. Black, white, Asian, it didn't matter, they were all one crowd. There were times when as many as eight or ten young people were eating lunch and exchanging lively repartee around the dining room table, many of them among the top students in their classes. These young people were wonderful friends and companions to each other throughout high school.

Our food budget seemed to reflect Don's job—it was astronomical! We had a pantry, fridge, and cabinets bulging with cereal, cookies, snacks, and drinks, all purchased from warehouses like Aldi's and Cub in an attempt to control the budget. Food was the hallmark of our hospitality. The kids and their friends came in the door and headed for the pantry. Most of the boys' friends were moderate in their consumption, but Paul was definitely a cookie monster. He would down several cookies with milk, and then, on his way out, he would slip a few more into his coat pocket. It was okay because Paul's mom Sarah did a lot of early-morning driving to swim team practice when I was unable to make the trip. Paul was welcome to all the cookies he wanted!

We never knew how many people we would be having for dinner. If the boys had friends in the house when dinnertime came, they were invited to stay. It was not uncommon to have nine or ten around the table for weekday evening meals. One young man named Kaz had a remarkable talent for ringing the doorbell just as we were sitting down to eat. Kaz was six feet tall, weighed about 200 pounds, and had a correspondingly prodigious appetite. He liked our food, but mostly he liked to just be in the family and know he was welcome.

Cooking the food and clearing up afterward was a huge, daily task that was shared by the whole family and supported by our housekeeper Dorothy, who came three times a week. We had a "Chart" that was taped on the kitchen wall with each person's daily duties clearly marked. Guests were not exempt from service—it was part of being family.

When people came into our home, they felt like it was a place they could relax and be comfortable. For years we had an old red sectional in the living room that seemed to invite both kids and adults to just curl up and fall asleep. Due to the swallowy soft cushions, it was a good place for hugging. Since the sectional was movable, I never knew what arrangement the living room would be in next. The kids would move the pieces around the room to accommodate participation in video games, video nights with popcorn, and, occasionally, a swim team party.

The swim team produced more heroic action by the York parents than any of the boys' other activities. Throughout their high school years, the family would rise at 5:15 a.m., and one of us, most frequently Don, would fix food for the day—three hot, portable breakfasts, three lunches, and three afternoon snacks—package them, and herd everyone out the door in time to get to a 6 a.m. swim practice! It was a drill we still remember with astonishment, shaking our heads and wondering how we did it.

Chlorine was the family perfume. Swim practices happened twice a day, and swim meets occupied nearly every weekend in the winter. Don and I, especially Don, were big swim team boosters, and we were at nearly every event. Don organized fundraising, transportation, and Christmas-break training trips. I coordinated events such as the annual "shaving" party, which occurred when the city swimming championships came around. The whole team would come over to our house and spend the day shaving off all the hair on their heads and bodies, abiding by the theory that shaving off the hair would help them shave seconds off their times. Our son Maurice, who was the fastest man on the team and who had a mane of gorgeous, long, wavy-black locks, would usually retain his hair as a statement that he was fast enough to flaunt it. The hair-shaving ritual became legendary when he was suspiciously disqualified on the start of his 50 meter free race at the city championships. He protested by shaving it all off before his next race. His bald head revved the team to an adrenaline high that carried them to a hard-fought win over their arch rivals. Thus, shaving took on the quality of a tribal bonding ritual, accompanied by body painting and a pow-wow accented by grunting, chanting and whooping. After it was over I usually had to call the plumber for hair removal from the drains.

I loved being "Mom." Since I rarely went out, my home was my palace. After the lonely years of my early illness, I enjoyed the companionship, the affirmations, and the feelings of fulfillment I experienced in having people feel comfortable and loved in my home. I felt that the most important thing Don and I were achieving during those years was holding the family together and giving the boys a rich, happy home life, even in the midst of my own physical distress and Don's strenuous daily output of energy to keep it all functioning. I was everybody's "Mom" throughout the years of my deepest illness.

The "Mom" persona lasted until my healing began to change my shape, size, appearance and personality. When I was soft, homey and a little overweight, everyone called me "Mom." Later, when I slimmed down to a somewhat athletic-looking 130 pounds, only my own boys would call me Mom. Even they, when they gave me a hug around my angular shoulders, would sometimes laughingly say, "Wow, Mom, where are you? Is it really you?"

Parking Violations

I was out for a swim at the YMCA, and, as frequently happened, I was cruising around the parking lot, trying to find a parking space. I insisted on going to the Y by myself, because it was the one regular independent act I could perform without getting into trouble—at least that's what Don thought! He didn't know I had secretly become a crusader for handicapped rights at the Y and that not everybody was appreciative of my efforts.

Swimming was not just the male form of family exercise, it was mine too. Since I couldn't stand on my feet, I got my exercise by swimming three times a week. My body's thermal regulation was askew, and I could not tolerate activity that made me too hot. The cool water in the pool not only cushioned my body but also moderated my body temperature so I could exercise my muscles. The activity produced good old endorphins in my brain that made me feel better. I had some of my best inspirations while swimming laps.

The big problem I had with swimming was access. I had to have a close parking space or I couldn't make the short walk into the locker room without getting all worn out. It was a feat I clung to stubbornly as a monitor three times a week that I could still do it. When the Y first opened, I had lobbied for handicap parking, had provided stickers for policing offenders and had protested loudly when unauthorized vehicles parked in the reserved spaces—a frequent offense. Sometimes I had to turn around and go home because I couldn't get into the building.

On this particular night, all three vehicles in the designated spaces were non-handicapped, and I was mad! I wasn't going to give up my swim. I cruised around a couple of times, and then I pulled my big old blue Oldsmobile station wagon right up to within three inches of the rear bumpers of the offending cars, blocking any possibility of their leaving the lot. I stopped the engine, removed the keys, grabbed my swim bag and exited the car, locking it behind me. Then I slowly made my way up the ramp with my cane and into the reception area. I asked to talk to the Director but was informed that he was "busy." "Okay," I thought, "we'll see about that." I sat down in the lobby and waited for the fireworks.

Ten minutes later, a full-figured woman in a full-length black leather coat with a spiky black fur collar pushed her way through the doors, eyes flashing and jaw set in an angry clench. She headed for the desk and stood there with one leather-gloved hand on her hip and the other on the counter, fingers tapping impatiently.

"May I help you," asked the clerk, eying the woman with caution.

"Some damn fool has parked his car behind mine in the lot, and I can't get out. I have an appointment to make, and I want that car moved!"

"Hmm," I thought. "Am I up to this?" I screwed my courage to the sticking point. I got up out of my chair, gripped my cane tightly in case I needed to use it for defense, and walked over to the counter. "Excuse me," I said, looking directly into the face of the angry woman and knowing the attendant was there to call security if the feline tried to claw through her leather gloves and scratch my eyes out. "I am the person who parked behind you. You parked in a handicapped space, and I couldn't get into the Y any other way."

Catwoman flexed her gloved hand and turned to the attendant. "Are you going to let her get away with that? Make her move her car!" She was almost shouting, and she was attracting the attention of other people in the lobby. The attendant's eyes were shifting back and forth between us, and she was looking anxious. Her hand was on the phone.

"Excuse me," I said to the attendant in a calm voice. "People are always parking in handicapped spaces and the Y is not doing anything about it. When I can't park, I have to go home. Please tell the Director that I want to meet with him."

"I'm sorry ma'am," she started, but I interrupted.

"I'm not going to move my car until he agrees." I raised my eyebrows, pursed my lips and stared at the young lady, then at the glaring Catwoman, who began to show her teeth and make small hissing sounds. I turned around and headed back to my seat.

"Do it!" Cat Woman snarled at the attendant and then began stalking up and down in front of me, her hair standing on end and her tail waving threateningly behind her. I sat down sedately, crossed my hands, closed my eyes, took a deep breath and feigned sleep. Five minutes later I was ushered into the Director's office, with Catwoman still stalking and staring holes through the door after me. I sat leisurely in the chair opposite the Director and made my case—and the case of a lot of other disabled people who had as much right as anyone else to use the facilities. Gradually the tension in his face relaxed and he broke into a grin. "Mrs. York, we'll take care of this. I'll have security check the lot regularly and ticket offenders."

"Thank you," I said. "I appreciate it. Would you like to start by having one of your men move my car and park it so Cat—er, ahem, excuse me—the lady outside can get her car out?"

"Sure thing."

Life at the Y was a lot easier after that, for me and a lot of other disabled folks.

The Man in My Life

A dream as big as the Universe, a heart as big as the sky. That's the man in my life.

I often remember that night my mother described to me so many years ago, the night when she was watching the stars with Don on the athletic field at the Boy Scout camp. After pointing out to her the various constellations and familiar stars, he waved his arm across the sky and said, "It's all mine." That statement turned out to be a prophetic one, one that has been fulfilled over the span of all our forty-five years together.

It began in 1966, when Don started graduate school in Astronomy at the University of Chicago. He went on from there to work for Princeton University, doing ground-breaking work with *Copernicus*, the first space telescope. Eventually, he returned to the University of Chicago as the Horace B. Horton Professor of Astronomy and Astrophysics. In the 1980's, he became the Founding Director of the first remotely controlled telescope, the 3.5 meter telescope at Apache Point in New Mexico. In the 1990's he served as the Founding Director for the Sloan Digital Sky Survey (SDSS), also located at Apache Point, a project designed to map a large portion of the Universe in great detail. SDSS has produced massive amounts of data that has transformed much of our understanding of the Universe. It has been one of the most successful astronomy projects ever built. Don has written hundreds of scientific papers and is listed among the top four scientists in the world with "hot" papers, according to a survey that tabulates the number of citations to scholarly work. In terms of his professional expertise, he is an awesome man. One of his favorite sayings, "Make no small plans," has been the hallmark of his career.

Many people can be a success professionally and be a failure in other aspects of their life and relationships. Not so with my man. The motivation for all his work comes from his profound sense of God's presence and calling in all that he does. There was a time early in his vocation when he was faced with a choice of whether to move forward in science or to go into social service. At an altar call one night in Virginia, he moved over to a far corner of the sanctuary and knelt to pray between the pews in the choir section, seeking God about which path he should take. As he quieted himself before God, he felt hands on both of his shoulders, even though no humans were anywhere near him. He saw his life pass before him and saw that God had prepared the way for him at every point of decision, opening the doors for him to receive the finest scientific education and preparation. He knew in his deepest heart that his work of serving God would be in science. From that moment, he never looked back. He pursued every project with energy that came not only from his own prodigious resources but also from a compelling sense of God's empowerment. The pursuit of excellence with a humble spirit defines his walk with God.

The fact that Don was committed to a scientific career focused on the heavens did not cut off the possibility of his serving people on the Earth. He discovered practical, down-to-earth uses for the massive data handling capacities developed by the Sky Survey. He established CUIP (Chicago Public Schools-University of Chicago Internet Project), which became the driving force for getting Internet service into 30 Chicago schools in the neighborhood of the University. The CUIP program included hard-wiring the schools, acquiring computers for every classroom, providing staff and workshops to train teachers, and developing interactive classroom materials for use by teachers. Don drew in participation by all of Chicago's museums and libraries in order to provide educational resources. His commitment and tenacity in fighting bureaucracies to get the work done made him much beloved by Principals and teachers in all of the CUIP schools. Once again, he made no small plans. In this case, his plans affected the quality of education for thousands of Chicago public school students, many of them in very poor neighborhoods.

Don's relationships also testify to his magnanimous heart. He insists that his students call him "Don"—not "Professor York"—and they love him for his kindness as well as his excellence. As for me, well, Don has always been and will always be my heart's true love, my companion in good and bad times, a faithful and loving father, a solid provider, a rock in the midst of the storm. When Don chose astronomy as his avocation, he chose well. It is, perhaps, the only stage expansive enough for him to express the largeness of his soul.

All the same, with all of his amazing qualities, Don is a human being who has not yet achieved a state of divine perfection. Sometimes that has been hard for me to accept. Through the years I have come to a firm belief that we were brought together by Providence in order that we might share refinement in the crucible of life. In order to come forth as gold, the impurities of our personalities must be purged out, a process that occurs through intense heat. Certainly the flame of suffering was turned up high in our lives. We have learned things together about life and about God that we could never have learned as separate individuals.

But the price of gold is high and the process of transformation is costly indeed. Perhaps it is only when the product comes through, pure and gleaming in the Sun, that we can know it was all worthwhile. When you're in the crucible, you just wish you could turn down the burner.

Don and I never did know how to have a good fight. There are several reasons for this. First of all, neither of us had any role models for fighting. We both came from gentle, soft-spoken folk who were more prone to serving others than fighting for their own way. Don's father died when he was young, so he didn't have any model of parents working out their conflicts. His mother is one of the sweetest souls on earth, and in all of my years of marriage to Don I have never heard her say a disparaging word about anyone. No conflict.

As for me, I grew up in a culture of harmony, not just on the surface, but deep down. I never heard my mother and father raise their voices at each other, nor was I aware of it if they ever had any serious conflicts. They each had their roles to play, my father doing the farm work or real estate work and my mother teaching and caring for the family, and they supported each other in these roles. Whenever there was a joint decision to be made, whether it was a big financial decision or a smaller matter of family discipline, my father and mother presented a united front and devoutly stuck with each other through whatever might come. It was only in their elderly years, when my father was around the house more than he was in his younger days, that I began to notice some irritation regarding television watching. My father enjoyed watching westerns, crime shows and sports, and he highly valued my mother's companionship for these viewing sessions. He would say, "Sit right here, Mommy, and watch this with me," and he would smile and wink at her. Mother did not like television, especially westerns, crime shows and sports, and she disliked being tied down in front of the TV. She preferred to be reading her Bible, writing, or preparing devotional tapes and materials. To keep the peace, and to "take care of Daddy," she would sit there and watch television with slightly pursed lips and little invisible fumes floating over her head.

Another reason Don and I didn't know how to fight is that for most of our marriage, amazingly, we were in agreement with each other. We had no reason to fight. We talked things through, came to understanding with each other, and made decisions we both supported. Don and I always gave each other space to do the things we wanted to do and the things we felt God wanted us to do. He was there with me through all my changes, from speaking in tongues to changing church denominations, and I was always there for him, supporting his work and travel, praying for him, believing God was working in him as he was doing his profession. Even when I experienced the pain and loneliness of his being away for several days a week, I accepted it as a necessary situation, at least for the time being.

We also had a deeply-held but unspoken belief that expressing one's own needs, and especially insisting on them, is selfish and, perhaps, un-Christian. If one is a mature Christian, the concern should be about other people's needs, not one's own. Of course, we each did fulfill our own personal needs, but those needs never really interfered seriously with the other person—not until progressively serious chronic illness set in. By that time we were deep into the self-deception that we could bury our own needs and feelings beneath a brave, godly appearance and that somehow the mask would become the reality.

The belief that the family was more important than anything else also kept us from airing and resolving our issues. Even when the stress became serious, after many years of disability and self-denial, we silently bore the pain because we wanted to maintain the semblance of "normalcy" at all costs. We often joked about living a "normal" life, because we certainly had no idea what "normal" was! We didn't display our marital laundry because it was tough enough that I was physically disabled; we didn't want the kids to see our deeper human frailties flying in the wind as well.

In spite of our valiant efforts at repressing our feelings, Don's job became a matter of increasing stress between us. As the Founding Director of two large, cutting-edge telescopes, he was able to envision extraordinary scientific projects and also to bring the resources and people together to nurture them into practical reality. But these projects didn't just miraculously appear on the mountain in New Mexico. They came to birth through extremely painful labor. Don was frequently gone for a few days every week. He would be up at five on Monday morning, dressed and heading out the door, and I would roll over, open one eye and say, "Where are you going?"

"I told you. I have to fly to Seattle for a meeting about funding. I'll be back Wednesday night, but I have to be out at Fermi for the next two days to talk about data reduction. Can you fix the boys' breakfast?"

"Mmm." I said as he pulled on his jacket, gave me a quick kiss and headed down the long hallway. I heard the click of the door at the other end. He said, "I told you—," but I often forgot where he was going or when he was coming back. It wasn't that he didn't make preparations as well as possible for his absence. He was always thoughtful and always laid the groundwork by having the fridge full of food and making sure other household needs were covered. It was just so hard to keep it all going! I tried to cover up how hard it was so he wouldn't feel bad about it. I thought I was pretty good at cover-ups.

When Don went out the door, I would roll over for a few minutes, getting myself ready for the morning drill: Wake the gang, make three hot breakfasts of eggs on English muffins, juice and fruit, and pack them in individual bags for each boy to eat after swim practice was over; label with names; pack three big lunches with sandwiches, fruit, juice, chips and a brownie; finally, bag up three after-school snacks with all the trimmings. A swim team travels on its stomach, and there were two practices a day—6:00 a.m. and 4:00 p.m. Fueling the swim tank was a daily challenge. Then there would probably be last-minute homework printouts and at least one other unanticipated crisis before all three boys bundled up in parkas and boots and hurried out the door. As I thought about the hectic hour ahead, I would brace myself, swing my feet over the side of the bed, slip on my sweatpants and sweatshirt, shift to my scooter and head for the kitchen, telling myself over and over, "I can do this. It's not that long, I can do it."

When Don was home, he was often up into the small hours of the morning, dealing with budgets and personnel issues. "Charlie," a recalcitrant but crucial employee at the mountain, was the bane of my life. It seemed like Don never stopped talking about Charlie. Charlie, Charlie, Charlie. Charlie this, Charlie that. Charlie in the bedroom, Charlie in the bathroom, Charlie in the office, Charlie at prayer meetings and at the dinner table. Charlie caused so much trouble I wished they could shoot him into outer space where they could conveniently view him through the telescope as a safely distant asteroid. If it wasn't Charlie it was Larry—or Anita or Burt. I was sick of phone calls that ran to one in the morning, I was sick of the trips, I was sick of what I saw it all doing to Don and what it was doing to us.

I found I couldn't "cover up" forever. About once every three months we had a "conversation," our way of clearing the air. That was about as frequently as it could happen, because the pressure was so intense that we had no space for daily airing. So I saved up my "issues" until I found an opportune moment. Unfortunately, it was usually on an evening when we carefully carved out a time to go out for dinner or for a short weekend. He would be looking forward to a rare relaxing evening, and I would be looking for a way to pull the cork on my bottled up emotions. There we would be, eating a nice meal and supposedly enjoying ourselves, and I would initiate the "conversation," knowing it might be my only chance until "who knows when." Suddenly a simple celebration would turn into an intense analysis session.

I discovered that males and females have different perspectives about expressing needs. For many women, and certainly for me, expressing emotions is a necessary outlet: "Why do you have to work so much! It's not good for you. Look, you're getting overweight. I'm so worried about you. And we never have any time together. I love you. What about our relationship? You don't listen to my poetry anymore." I would release the emotion, then I would feel better, the moment would pass, and I would forget about it. Not so with men—at least not with my man. As a deeply compassionate person, Don would listen carefully to my feelings and keep meticulous tabs on everything I said. He is also an intellectual and scientific man, and he was fatally inclined to indulge the fantasy that masculine reasoning will prevail over feminine emotion. He would present all of his logical reasons why I should not feel the way I did. Enticed by the assumed superiority of the rational over the emotional and intuitive, I would attempt to move my feelings over into the realm of reason, an enterprise somewhat akin to harnessing the wind in a handbag. All it did was make me angrier. Anger made me feel guilty, and guilt made me work that much harder to squelch my "un-Christian" passions lest they imperil my immortal soul. There was a hymn we sang frequently when I was young: "Angry words, O let them never from the tongue unbridled slip." As hard as I tried, the horses slipped those bridles all too frequently.

The burden of our situation was enough to sink any normal man, but Don was not a normal man! Most men with wives like me would have been long gone. Divorce statistics are high for people with MS. Even with his generous heart, his prodigious strength and his indomitable will, however, Don began to show signs of the struggle. He began to interpret my feelings as an ultimatum, a law that must be followed, a dictum to be obeyed. I became an unwitting dictator. The burden of things that had to be done, supposedly to meet my demands, eventually became very heavy, even for him, and he began to have a weary countenance, visibly suffering from the load he was bearing. I felt guilty and ashamed that I caused him so much trouble, and he felt guilty for not taking good care of me. All the guilt was like old dirty oil, clogging our carburetor. Our engine began to go out of tune. He couldn't see letting go of projects he had started, and I thought that in that case he should not start so many new ones. I stopped feeling that his work was his divine calling and began feeling it was a personal compulsion that was detrimental our lives and health. We grew apart.

It all came to a head one evening when I was sitting in the Chicago Theatre at a performance of *Riverdance* with an empty seat beside me. We had decided to "do something nice" for ourselves, and we got tickets for three of us months in advance so Don could clear his schedule. I allowed myself to anticipate the event a little too much. Unfortunately, Don had to make an emergency trip to Washington the same day, and there was a heavy fog whiting out the airport when he was due to come in. He called from Washington and said he would meet us at the theatre. Jeremy got me there, handled my electric scooter, and broke the trail to the reserved handicap seats. When the show started and Don wasn't there, I was worried at first, and then I became angry. I sat there fuming at the same time I was trying to enjoy the show. So why couldn't he make it to a special date set up months in advance! He had time for everyone but me!

About a half hour into the first act Don showed up apologizing. I heard the mumbled explanation of a bad flight, etcetera, and turned back to the stage, determined to enjoy myself. After the intermission, however, I got really ticked off when, despite the clicking heels of about a hundred energetic dancers on the stage, he nodded off to sleep and slept through most of the fabulous show that was supposed to be such a special evening for us. So much for romance!

It was a few weeks later, in early 1995, when we learned that Don's precipitous weight gain and tendency to fall asleep at any moment was due to high blood pressure and diabetes. The stress in his life—and mine—had finally caught up with him—and us. I was extremely worried about him. First I felt scared, then I felt guilty, and then I became angry again. Why hadn't he heard me when I expressed my concerns! But now that Don and I were both ill, we had even less space to release the emotional pressure. Later on, during my healing process, I would discover that I had repressed my emotions for many years and that this repression contributed to my illness. It wasn't Don's fault. It was just my nature—and his—and both of ours together. We were not only dealing with extremely difficult life circumstances but also deeply ingrained personal characteristics that were part of our family heritage and our gender identities.

Looking back on it, there were a lot of things we didn't do well at all, but there were some things we did very well indeed. We did not become one of those MS divorce statistics. We managed to raise a wonderful family, all of our boys growing up to be gentle, kind, compassionate human beings. Eventually, through all the struggles, Don and I would have to seriously confront and acknowledge the need for healing our emotions and our relationship. In that process, we would discover something holding our marriage together that is deeper than passion, deeper than suffering, deeper than all the troubles life can bring our way. At that time, however, we didn't have the clairvoyance to look into the future and see that things would turn out okay. The heat was turned up high, and the crucible was a most uncomfortable place to be.

Flashes in My Soul

People do not usually die from multiple sclerosis, but it sometimes happens that people become critically paralyzed or that their lives are cut short from complications of the disease. Shanta was the first one to sense what seemed to him to be the inevitable but drawn-out approach of my death. Trained not only as a pastor but also as a hospital chaplain, he assessed my deteriorating situation as being so serious that he came to my home to help prepare me to die.

I remember the pain of that meeting in 1994. We sat in the back sunroom, I in the orange recliner and he on a straight chair facing me. We had become friends over a period of five years, making contact almost daily about various ministry issues in the church, and I had shared my struggles with him. On this day his eyebrows were drawn together at the center and his forehead was wrinkled in concern. His eyes were full of both pain and compassion. He leaned over with his elbows on his knees, took my hands and said in a husky voice, "Shall we pray?" I nodded, sensing that the words to come were too weighty to be spoken in any medium other than prayer. He began to pray, saying, "God, thank you so much for Anna and the blessing she is to everyone who knows her. Thank you for giving her a mighty portion of your Spirit and courage to face all the challenges she has each day. God, today I have a burden on my heart, and I hope you will help me with this." He paused and seemed to struggle for words. My heart stopped as I entered into a timeless space in which I would hear with my soul. He began haltingly, "God, every one of us has a certain time here on earth. I pray that you will help Anna as she faces the reality of her situation. Help her to never give up hope and to always look to you. Also, Lord, if it is necessary, I pray you would help her prepare to come to you when it is time to do so. Help us to all be with her as she faces whatever will happen."

As he prayed, tears began to flow down and drop on his hands. As I heard him in that eternal moment and understood what he was say-

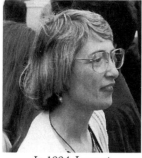
In 1994, I was at my lowest point.

ing, it registered as truth in my own heart. Yes, it seemed that's the way things could go. It might be a long time, but it might not be. I needed to start now, while I still had just a little strength, to face the challenge for my family and myself. Shanta, as a true friend, was trying to help me. I also began to weep softly, a gentle, purging rain, cleansing my doubts, strengthening my courage and resolve, preparing me for the task ahead. He finished praying and then looked in my tear-stained face, giving my hand a gentle squeeze. "Anna, this is very difficult for me, but as your pastor and your friend, I need to help you come to grips with this."

Others in my circle of intimacy also felt I was fading quickly. Early in 1995, several members of our small group had dreams in which children died and were then resurrected or resuscitated. In my own dream, there was a very small, seemingly dead child in a glass box, and I blew into the box vigorously, trying to revive her. In the next scene the child was larger, and I was holding her close to me giving her mouth-to-mouth resuscitation. It seemed that I was the child. Two women dreamed of my death, and one dreamed three times of my death and resurrection. We prayed for insight and understanding about what God was saying to us. The theme of resurrection began to permeate all the melodies of my heart as I longed for release from my pain.

Scott, one of the Catholic members of our group, brought me a very special gift, a copy of the works of St. Theresa of Avila. Since I was raised as a Protestant—and a conservative one—I had no acquaintance with the great saints and mystics of the church; thus, I had no context or reference point for the spiritual experiences I was having during the years of my illness. It was as though I was a lonely pioneer on the spiritual frontier, trying to forge my own tools to build my spiritual house, work my fields, and gather in my own crops. I had no idea that there were other people with similar experiences who had gone before me and paved the way by developing disciplines of prayer and meditation and by describing the spiritual journey they took in pain and faith. I did not realize my utter destitution. I did not know I had been re-inventing the spiritual wheel.

When I opened the covers of Theresa's collected works I suddenly found myself in fellowship with a soul who was closer than a sister—indeed, I felt that I was meeting my very own self. Theresa and I fellowshipped deeply and intimately. She opened my own experience to me, giving me perspective, helping me identify myself as one who is not alone but who is in company with many others who have trod a similar path throughout the ages. Theresa, like me, had a serious chronic illness that sounded somewhat like mine. In her fiftieth year, she recovered, and after that she wrote most of her major works. I noted that it was now my fiftieth year.

Theresa introduced me to St. John of the Cross. Through him I discovered the "dark night of the soul" and was able to understand that I had experienced the dark night of the soul in the classical sense he described, and, indeed, I had been in it for thirteen years!

Through John and Theresa I increasingly understood my suffering as an integral part of my path to God, a purification of my soul. Whereas I had already come to a place of peace regarding my illness, a feeling that I was completely in the arms of Christ, I moved on to the hope that my experience was preparing me for an even deeper relationship, a whole new dimension of union with the resurrected Christ.

The hope, and even the expectation of this possibility, was enhanced by a "vision" of the resurrected Christ that changed my life in powerful, practical ways. I saw the risen Christ, vibrant and healthy, meeting me in a relaxed and friendly way, somewhat as a husband might meet his spouse at the dinner table at the end of the day. He showed me a table full of every kind of food one can imagine, prepared exquisitely, a banquet beyond what the human mind can imagine, with food from many nations and cultures. We sat down, and he put his elbows on the table and looked into my face. With a gentle smile, he said, "What shall we eat?"

I looked at the table and was overwhelmed. I didn't even know what most of the foods were, and I had no idea which ones would suit me or which ones might be good for me. I decided he would know better than I, so I turned to him and said, "What do you suggest?"

With an expansive smile and with great joy, he answered, "I will give you myself. I am your bread!" It seemed like a fire kindled within me and a flame of love ignited me. Images of manna, bread, and the Last Supper flashed into my mind. I reached out my arms and said, "Yes! Yes! That's what I want! I want nothing but you." I saw the cross in the background, but the risen Christ was between the cross and me. I was enveloped with his living, breathing, resurrected Presence.

My encounter with Christ opened me even more to the hope and expectation that I would come into a place of union with Christ. I could envision myself being with him as a friend and companion, and possibly even as a spouse, in the classical, mystical sense. This hope transformed suffering from something that must be borne to the possibility of offering it as a gift to my beloved, an expression of my deepest commitment to purify and prepare myself for union with him. I knew he would receive my gift and wear it as a gem.

I have tried you
But not as silver
In the furnace
I have chosen you
So my delight may be
In your purity
And your gold may be a crown
Upon my wounded brow
A precious diadem
By which you honor me
A gem I wear to honor you
With my love

The deeper my identification with Christ, the more I began to experience "flashes" in my soul. They were flashes of glory that were the more brilliant because my suffering was so deep.

Whence come these flashes in my soul,
Like holy fire from God's own throne,
Searing, wounding me with love
All consuming me with love?
What exquisite pain
To bear this flame.

I began to think of Christ as "my beloved." We shared a very tender relationship in which I was assured of his unconditional love. Passages in the Song of Solomon became deeply meaningful to me: "I am my beloved's and he is mine. He brought me to his banqueting table. His banner over me was love."

The more I experienced being loved and desired unconditionally, even in my weak and broken condition, the more I was able to open myself in my innermost being to be filled with Christ's life. At the same time he was desiring me, he was also empowering me to be his own beloved.

While I did not know what was to come or how it would come, I had a strong sense that I would be physically as well as spiritually changed. I had a sense of active waiting for a transformation of my whole being. In my dreams I would skip lightly, barely touching the earth, "leaping upon the mountains" and "bounding over the hills."

The tender relationship with Christ changed my view of myself. Whereas I had previously felt that Christ was completely the giver and I the receiver, I began to experience more mutuality, as though I had something incredibly precious to offer to Christ and that I could offer it with joyous freedom because he would receive it with joy. My meditations were full of the imagery of gardens. I felt that Christ would come into my innermost being as into a garden that had been carefully tended and prepared for many years. We would eat and rejoice together in the fullness and abundance of life. I had the sense that as we shared life together Christ would show me new horizons in the spirit. I asked and expected that Christ would introduce me to his friends and show me the way in the spiritual realm. I was confident that I could explore with no fear whatever because I could know with absolute assurance from that time on that we were completely joined. I was fully protected and Christ would never allow anything but good to happen to me.

My experience of union with Christ was accompanied by a powerful yearning for my own resurrection. The Rising Spirit that was born and bred in me through generations and that had grown stronger and stronger as I nourished it in prayer and meditation was rising up in me. I had experienced a spiritual rising, and now I wanted a physical rising. I longed to be free to love and serve with no physical hindrance. I had a hope and expectation that I would rise to be with and be like Christ. I imagined what it would be like and wrote some anthems that called for rising up to greet Christ's Resurrection day, for rising up to be set free from all human limitations. I envisioned my body as being filled with light and rising with Christ. I connected my own longing for rising to a larger, cosmic need for transformation of the created world, which also longed to be released into new liberty.

In retrospect, there is no doubt in my mind that Christ was preparing me for a Rising. I thought at that time that it would take me out of my physical body and into a new spiritual body like Christ's, into a sphere of service free of human limitation. I didn't know Christ had in mind that my Rising would heal and rejuvenate my physical body so that I could live in a new dimension of health and wholeness as Anna York on planet Earth.

Rising UP!

Jubilee!

It was my fiftieth birthday, October 27, 1995, and I had not yet made the expected trip to meet my Maker. In fact, I was riding a horse! Don and I were in French Lick in the rolling hills of southern Indiana at the height of the autumn Indian summer glory. French Lick was once famous for its mineral springs and served as the watering hole for Presidents and other famous people from around the world. The old hotel has been restored, and there are golf courses, trails, and riding stables. I was feeling enough energy that I decided on my birthday to go for a horseback ride. It was a wild idea for one such as me, but I knew the horses on the ranch would do nothing but walk. I wanted to see the autumn colors and explore trails I could not reach on my scooter.

Don was horrified at the idea. Nevertheless, he and Jerry, a burly stable hand, helped me mount up. They put a bale of hay next to Daisy, a droopy-headed old sorrel, and Don supported me while Jerry lifted my left foot and placed it in the stirrup. Then he steadied me while Don got his shoulder under my derrière and gave a big boost. When I was up high enough, leaning over the horn of the saddle and grabbing it with both hands, I shifted my right leg over to the other side and slowly came somewhat erect in the saddle. I felt pretty dizzy up there for a moment and had strong second thoughts about the whole escapade. Don, a born and bred city kid and completely unacquainted with equines, was looking really worried.

"What if he starts to run?" he asked.

Jerry raised his eyebrows as though that was a highly amusing idea and shook his head. "Naw, that horse ain't runnin' nowhere. She ain't run anywhere for years. She'll just follow old Red real slow."

Don wasn't convinced. I adjusted my position in the saddle and said, "See honey? It's just like riding in a car!"

As it turns out, getting on the horse was probably the biggest challenge of the event. My horse was the slowest, dullest nag this side of the Rio Grande. She ambled off down the trail with her nose at the tail of the preceding horse and never looked up for the rest of the trip. Don drove back and forth on the upper road in the van, trying to keep me in sight at all times to be sure the old plug didn't throw me or that I didn't fall off. No sweat. The back of that horse was as broad as an easy chair! I was exhausted when I was finished, but incredibly happy. I had done an exploit, a sure sign of Jubilee.

The idea of Jubilee comes from the ancient Jewish tradition that time should be marked in 50-year blocks and that in the fiftieth or "Jubilee" year all slaves should go free, all debts that had accumulated in the previous forty-nine years should be forgiven and all ancestral lands that had been sold for debt should return to their original owners. Jubilee was a powerful expression that conditions of human pain, injustice and inequity are only temporary and that God intends liberation for all people. Some of my friends had love and faith enough to declare that my 50th birthday would be the beginning of a year of "Jubilee"—a year in which I would be set free.

There were some signs of new possibilities. I had been on Betaseron, a new drug for MS, for about a year. Betaseron was the first drug that could actually affect the course of the disease, and my neurologist was one of the leading researchers. I responded to the drug in a statistical fashion—one of the few times in my life I have complied with statistics!—experiencing less frequent and less severe episodes of MS. There was no way of knowing for sure, of course, whether my apparent progress was just another blip on my disease monitor or whether it was a sign of sustained recovery. Anyway, I was able to do a little walking with a cane, although I still used my scooter most of the time.

Jubilee was also in evidence in the big changes I had made in my diet. I had had time to reflect on my encounter with Christ at the banqueting table. At that time I had heard Christ saying the words "simple food." When I asked, "What is simple food?" I saw several kinds of food in front of me, including vegetables, grains, fruits, and fish with scales. Apparently, among all the culinary possibilities available to me, I was to choose healthier fare. A short time after that, Sean, my oldest son, presented me with Roy Laver Swank's *Multiple Sclerosis Diet Book* and said, "Mom, you need to read this." Other people had given me books about diet, but they had made no sense to me and I never followed through with any changes. Sean, however, was family. His exhortation, along with the banquet table experience, made me decide that it was now time to pay attention. Following Swank's lead, I immediately gave up eating red meat and began exploring ways to change the rest of my diet to meet the new criteria. I did not know it at the time, but the change in diet was to be the linchpin in my coming healing. It was the harbinger of a new jubilee world opening before me.

Jubilee was also happening for me in our church. People were beginning to express their conviction that I was engaged in pastoral work and that I was called to be a pastor. By the time my Jubilee birthday arrived, the idea of my being a pastor was gathering momentum, propelled by the love we shared in the community and acknowledgement of the grace in me that was touching many other lives. Shanta and other leaders in the church were in conversation about what it would mean for me to fulfill a pastoral calling in the context of our church.

I had a lot of fears. My health was so fragile that I feared I would get involved in serious ministry situations and disappoint everyone when my strength failed. Everyone might have to stop what they were doing to take care of me, resulting in embarrassment and frustration. What would happen to the people to whom I was ministering if I became ill—or died! Aren't pastors supposed to be strong and subordinate their personal needs to those of others? I needed a lot of help myself.

Stress was a big concern. I had been around churches long enough to know that politics, personal agendas, interpersonal conflicts, divisive arguments over doctrine, and backbiting against ministers were facts of life in most congregations. What if, for some reason I could not imagine, some of the people turned against me? Would I be able to bear it? Such a situation might send me into a tailspin worse than the one I was already in.

I also saw myself as being extremely vulnerable in ministry situations because all of it occurred in my home—since I didn't go out, people came in to see me. What if they came in and stayed too long, or refused to leave, or what if I had to ask them to leave? What about men coming into my home while I was alone? The thought of having to deal with such issues was daunting. After prayer and consultation with other leaders, I decided that I would not receive any males into my home unless another person was present, nor would I minister to any males unless another person was present.

I was concerned about my qualifications for ministry. Even though I had been doing ministry for most of my life, I didn't have the stamp of approval, the Master of Divinity degree that would validate me in the eyes of the larger world. Would people accept me as qualified without this degree? Some denominations have the degree as a requirement for ministry, but in the Baptist tradition individual churches are "autonomous," which means each church makes its own policies independently of any larger denominational authority. Baptist churches have always been free to determine the qualifications of their ministers, relying on observation of God's "anointing" on the person and the person's service within the church. Our church had several people with "M.Divs" in it. Would they approve a person who did not have the same qualifications as themselves? Besides that, one of the first pieces of chatter among newly-introduced clergy is, "And where did you go to school?" It's a piece of information that helps get people into categories so they can make associations— "Oh, I know so and so from there," etc. So what would I say? I remembered the conversation-stopping answer I gave back in Princeton when people asked, "So what do you do?" and I replied, "I'm a housewife." How would I feel about saying, "Well, I've been handicapped for years, and I don't have an M.Div." Coming into ministry without a degree seemed a little like going to a party naked—somewhat like the man in Jesus' parable who came into the wedding without a wedding garment on and was asked to leave. I was worried about going to the pulpit "naked." Where did I fit into the larger scene? What other people thought about me was one thing—how I would feel about myself was another.

Of all my fears, questions and concerns, the biggest was the definition of pastoral ministry. My ideas of pastoral ministry were all defined by traditional, male-dominated stereotypes. It seemed to me that even the women I observed ministering in Protestant churches were ministering according to masculine rules in a masculine paradigm. According to this paradigm, pastoral ministry is by its nature institutional and outward—a matter of expending a great deal of energy "doing" specific tasks in the church and in the outer world. Women at that time had such a hard time breaking through into any ministry that they were compelled to function according to the old masculine standards. Only in the Catholic church can one find more contemplative orders that would match my gifts—and I was not Catholic.

I did not fit into the masculine pastoral world. I did not have the strength to go around visiting people in their homes or in hospitals; I did not have the stamina to do administrative tasks or coordinate ministries throughout the community; I did not have the energy to preach. These "doing" activities did not fit with my brand of ministry, which was home based, personal, and inward, a matter of "being" with people and helping them "become," a matter of bringing new things into outward reality through the inward work of intercession and prayer. If I became a pastor, would I have to give up the inner work I was doing and take up outward tasks that were so foreign to me now? I didn't see how that would be possible with my disabilities. Besides, why would I want to give up something as incredibly fulfilling as the ministry I was currently doing?

It was the old "doing-being" dilemma with a new face on it. Now I was no longer entrenched in *doing* and struggling to find a way to *be*; I was firmly rooted in *being* and didn't know what it would be like to *do*! The pendulum of doing and being had swung completely opposite from where I began! How could a disabled female be a pastor? If Jubilee was coming, I wasn't sure what it would be like to be "free" and I didn't know if I would like it when it happened.

I Am Who I AM: Preparing for Ordination

There is a lot of fabulous computer software available today, and more amazing programs are being created every day. When new software is created, it often requires those who want to use it to do a system upgrade. I was new software. Shanta, the senior pastor of our church was the person who had the courage and initiative to upgrade our church "system" to make it work.

Shanta is from Sri Lanka, a strife-ridden country in which Christians are a small minority among the predominantly Buddhist population. His grandfather, also a Baptist pastor, was converted from Buddhism after being an ardent persecutor of Christians, providing Shanta with a powerful role model for changing paradigms. Shanta has seen firsthand the downsides of Christian proselytism in Asia and its links to Western cultural imperialism, and, as a result, he has a prophetic streak that denounces cultural cover-ups to the core message of the gospel. His Ph.D. in Religion from Northwestern gives him a comfortable breadth of theological perspective on Christianity in the context of a global culture.

Shanta is what many people would call a "radical." He challenges old definitions and works at creating new ones. He is especially ardent in fighting for economic and social justice, and his passion and prophetic leadership earned him renown in the Chicago Metropolitan region and around the country. Eventually, Shanta's leadership skills would earn him the position of Associate General Secretary for Interfaith Relations for the National Council of Christian Churches, and, later, the Executive of Inter-religious Dialogue and Cooperation for the World Council of Churches, a position he holds today. Remarkably, his work in the broader world does not distract his pastor's heart from attending to the sheep in his flock. While pastoring our church, he compassionately tended to people's needs, especially those who were downtrodden, oppressed or discriminated against in any way. I fit those categories for him—female, chronically ill, disabled. Besides that, we were friends, and we had been through a lot together. Shanta became a trailblazer for me.

Shanta recognized that the accepted roles of pastors conform to patriarchal models developed over millennia in a patriarchal church. We wrestled with what it would mean to break through these patriarchal definitions and get to a modern definition of pastoring that includes marginalized people such as women and the disabled. Trying to break through the patriarchal system was like trying to play a CD-ROM on an old IBM 286 from the 1970's. The system was seriously out of date and in need of an upgrade. We were a Southern Baptist Church at that time and were bucking the trend of suppressing women in the denomination. Southern Baptists are the largest protestant denomination in the country, with around 42,000 churches (more than the Catholics) and nearly 5000 missionaries—which means there are around 50,000 official ministry positions in the denomination. Within that context in the last thirty years approximately 1700 women have been ordained, but only about 200 women have held the position of Pastor or Co-Pastor. Our little congregation was already renegade in this regard. We had not only ordained two women but had also called a woman pastor who had guided our congregation for seven years before Shanta's arrival. Now we were wondering how a *disabled* female could fit into the picture.

We decided that our Baptist heritage had its downsides but also its upsides. Baptists have a tradition of congregational autonomy, which means each congregation can make its own policies and decisions. We also thought our smallness was an advantage—we were few in number, but our people were insightful and flexible enough to be open to change. We decided that change happens one person at a time and one church at a time. I was one person and ours was one church.

We looked at modern definitions of pastors. Those definitions say pastors have to have M.Divs, be chief executive officers, program coordinators, community activists, psychologists—Jacks (not Jills) of all trades. All of this besides going out and "saving the lost." Shanta and I called this the "role" model of pastoring—defining pastoring in terms of people who are qualified or "gifted" to fulfill specific roles. I didn't fit this paradigm at all.

In contrast, we discussed what we called the "person" model of pastoring, as described in the book of Ephesians. The Apostle Paul says that there are some people whom Christ gives as gifts to the church. These people are apostles, prophets, pastors, evangelists and teachers. These individuals are gifts in and of themselves, by virtue of who they are and what God has done in them. Their "work" is described in general terms as equipping the saints for the work of ministry, building up the body of Christ, and bringing people to maturity, to the "full stature of Christ." It says in general what they will do, but how they will do it is left open.

Shanta decided that I am a person whom Christ is giving to the church. As such, I am who I am—not who someone else is, and not what someone else does. It is my unique nature, it is "Who I AM" that is the gift. "Who I AM," meaning that my life, integrally joined with that of I AM, will build up the body of Christ in the ways and at the times I AM decides to do it. I settled it in my heart that I would *be* and *do* fine as long as I am God's person being "Who I AM."

Shanta was creating new software, new ways of thinking about ministry and church. The big task would be to find system compatibility in our church community. Shanta set about to create that compatibility by exploring and proposing changes in the structure of our church, changes that would enfranchise not just me but also others whose ministry had not been able to function in the outdated system.

Riding the Wind, Serving Tea: Ordination

It was January 17, 1997. I sat in my special reclining chair on the front row of our small church sanctuary and looked around at the beloved faces of those who had gathered for my ordination. Dhilanthi was playing her own wonderful arrangement of my song, "Coming Together," causing the spirit of it to flow out into the room and fill it with a special unity of love. The air was charged with blessing. Each person who took my hand looked directly into my eyes as though saying, "Yes, this is God's time for you." They all knew what an extraordinary event it was for me, a disabled woman, to be ordained to ministry in a Baptist church.

My dear friends from the congregation had worked hard to prepare the program. The evening was to be full of original music, beautifully arranged for voice, guitar and keyboards, by those who were touched by the creative stream of the Spirit that had been flowing through our church for a few years. Those on the worship team had carefully prepared their own songs and had also learned several of mine for the occasion. They were dressed festively and embraced me warmly with their smiles. They had received my ministry, believed in me, encouraged me and helped bring this occasion to fulfillment. Four of the families, those at the core of our small group, lovingly presented me with a sterling pendant of a shepherd carrying a lamb in her arms. On this evening my triumph was their own.

Friends and neighbors were there from all parts of our lives in the community, including a "stellar" group from Don's Astronomy Department at the University of Chicago. Don, who was stationed at the door, was deeply touched as, one after another, several senior members of the Department came in, greeted him and took their seats. Usually such distinguished scientists would only come together for a scientific function. To have them all in the church for my ordination was not only an honor but also a mark of their friendship. Later, we noted that all of those who had been chairman of the Astronomy

Department for the previous two decades were present, most of them with their wives.

Members of my ordination council were present. They were pastors from the area who had interviewed me to determine the appropriateness of my calling and had recommended me for ordination to our church. Among these was Susan Lockwood, who was pastor of our church prior to Shanta. She had endured the persecution of the Illinois Baptist Association, which had tried to eject our congregation from its ranks for calling a female as pastor. She was a remarkable, trail-blazing woman who helped prepare the way for women such as myself to do ministry. I was proud that she would give the ministerial charge after the official ordination.

One corner of the sanctuary was occupied by Dorothy Larkin's family. Dorothy had been my housekeeper for nearly a decade. She originally came to us as a "gift" when the University gave us a grant of money to aid us during a time of extreme suffering. Dorothy was indeed God's special gift to us, a loving, faithful, singing, praying woman who filled our house with the Holy Spirit each time she entered the door. I had invited Dorothy to give the invocation, and she had brought her family, including her husband and several grown sons and daughters, to celebrate the occasion. Their voices provided a reverent chorus of amens throughout the evening.

My sister had brought my 86-year-old father to Chicago so that he could confer his blessing on my ordination—his daughter!—a minister! It was a long way he had come, not just in miles. His personal study of scripture, in contradiction to his own upbringing and conservative church context, convinced him that females should be able to minister and "prophesy" because they have received the outpouring of the Spirit just the same as males. He was present at my ordination to take action on his convictions and convey his love and blessing for my ministry. His presence there represented to me the blessing and validation of all the preceding generations of godly ministers in my family, all the way back to Jamestown. I felt the presence of my Grandpa Horace Hinds, my beloved Grandma Anna Goforth Hinds, and my mother, who was too ill to come. I knew that my sister Ruth was there in spirit, although the trip from Oregon was too far for her to be physically present. My sister, Peggy Davis, would read my father's blessing and present family greetings to the congregation.

All four of our sons were there, and they had put together a quartet to sing a favorite family hymn, "It Is Well with My Soul." We had all lived this song together and it was like a healing balm when their voices blended in harmony:

When peace like a river attendeth my way,
When sorrows like sea billows roll;
Whatever my lot, Thou has taught me to say,
It is well, it is well with my soul.

And then, of course, there was Shanta. During the previous year, Shanta had broken with the old paradigm of single-pastor leadership and had led the church in the creation of a new pastoral team. The church's recognition of my calling to ministry had motivated a great deal of communal soul searching. We discovered other people within the church who were also doing pastoral ministry and wanted to empower and enfranchise them to do their work. The pastoral team concept was created, discussed, passed by the deacons, and approved by the church. It was a new way of thinking about church. Shanta had been teaching for years that every person in the church is a minister. According to him, a pastoral team of four persons was not coming into existence to pastor the members of such a small church. It was coming into existence to equip the members as ministers and to release the power of the Holy Spirit in them to reach out to a neighborhood of 50,000 and a city of 3.5 million. It was a bold vision, a bold step. Four of us were installed as a Pastoral Team in an official ceremony in November of 1996, just a few weeks prior to my ordination. The pastoral team installation and my ordination were the two crowning events of my Jubilee year. Indeed, I was being set free.

The evening of my ordination held many highlights that I will never forget, but the most significant for me, in retrospect, was Shanta's address. He told two stories that were destined to become parables of the new life of healing and transformation that was already opening before me.

The first was the story of a learned woman who read everything she could find and traveled the world seeking the meaning of life but could never find the answer. Some people told her they had heard of a man who had the answer but did not know where to find him. She searched in every country until finally, deep in the Himalayas, someone told her how to reach his house—a tiny little hut perched on the side of a mountain, just below the tree line. She climbed and climbed through the cold, craggy mountains until she reached the door, and then gathered her courage to knock.

"Yes?" said the kind looking old man who opened the door.

She thought she would die of happiness. "I have come halfway around the world to ask you one question," she said, gasping for breath. "What is the meaning of life?"

"Please come in and have some tea," the old man said.

"No," she said. "I mean, no thank you. I didn't come all this way for tea. I came for an answer. Won't you tell me, please, what is the meaning of life?"

"We shall have some tea," the old man said and started off toward the kitchen. The woman had no alternative but to come inside. While the tea was brewing she caught her breath and began to tell him about all the books she had read, about all the people she had met and about all the places she had been. The old man listened (which was just as well, since his visitor did not leave any room for him to reply), and as she talked he placed a fragile teacup in her hand. Then he began to pour the tea.

She was so busy talking that she did not notice when the teacup was full, and the old man just kept pouring until the tea ran over the sides of the cup and spilled to the floor in a steaming waterfall. "What are you doing?" she yelled when the tea burned her hand. "It's full, can't you see that? Stop! There's no more room!"

"Just so," said the old man with a faint smile. "You came here wanting something from me, but what am I to do? There is no more room in your cup. Come back when it is empty and then we'll talk."

Shanta followed this story immediately with one about a man named Nicodemus, who came to Jesus seeking the meaning of life. Jesus told Nicodemus, "No one can see the kingdom of God without being born from above." It was like Jesus poured tea all over Nicodemus' hand. Nicodemus protested, "How can anyone be born after having grown old? Can one enter into the mother's womb and be born?" He was saying, "Rabbi, my cup is full of tangible knowledge, religious knowledge too, and those are the only tools I have to understand what you are talking about—but it doesn't make sense!"

Nicodemus thought he knew all the answers, but something was missing. He knew there were signs, but he could not decode them. He wanted a straight answer from Jesus, a password that would unscramble the signal. Instead, the teacher invited him to take a plunge. "Believe in me—lean your whole life on me. Turn your cup upside down. Turn your mind inside out. Step out into the air. The wind blows wherever it pleases. You hear its sound, but you cannot tell where it comes from or where it is going. So it is with everyone born of the Spirit. Ride the wind, Nicodemus. Be born anew, Nicodemus."

Shanta went on to liken me to the man who was pouring the tea. He said that when he came to visit me, I poured tea for him and he would receive a new way to think about an issue, a new insight about himself, a new paradigm about the church or the world that came from my mystical, "being" nature. He said I was one of those people of prayer, people who listen to God, people who learn to trust God such that they are able to step out in faith and "ride the wind." He described how the church had been challenged during the last year to empty its cup and struggle with ways to open up possibilities for those who have unusual expressions of pastoral ministry, such as me.

He described how the church's "emptying the cup and letting it get filled again" had resulted in the formation of a "new thing," a Pastoral Team.

Shanta ended his address with these words: "We have learned—Anna has taught us more than anyone else—to put our busywork aside and "be" in God's presence. She has taught us to put our easy answers aside and fill our cups with Jesus' answers, to read the signs and be open to the new things God is doing among us. She has taught us—perhaps more than anyone else—to ride the wind, to be open to the leading of the Holy Spirit. So today, we ordain her. And in doing so, we affirm what God is doing in her, praise God for what God is doing in us through her, and we offer her as our gift to the church universal and the world at large. Today, Jesus says the same thing to us that he said to Nicodemus. 'Be born again, Nicodemus! Ride the wind! Come have a cup of tea!'"

The evening ended with individual blessings and prayers by those in the congregation, filing past, grasping my hands warmly and whispering sweet encouragement while heavenly music filled the air.

Among all the family, friends and church members who were there at my ordination, one group of people stood out as being unusual. They were members of the Tai Chi class I had been attending for about a year, including Sifu Bruce Moran. I had been telling my church about them for several months, but this was their first encounter with each other. As the Tai Chi people filed past to offer their blessings, some heads turned to get a better look. Who were these people? The strangers at my ordination were a sign that I was indeed riding the wind and that I would soon be pouring tea that would overflow many teacups.

Waving Palms: Healed by a Tai Chi Master

Now let's back up a few months to find out how those Tai Chi people were at such an unlikely event as my ordination. It was Palm Sunday of my Jubilee year, several months prior to my ordination, and I was at Tai Chi class on the University of Chicago campus. I had been coming to class somewhat sporadically for a couple of months. I was sitting on the back row of the class on a little folding stool, waving my arms more or less in the same fashion as everyone else, except I was sitting and they were standing. Occasionally I would stand for a couple of minutes to do an exercise, but I would wear out quickly and sit back down again. My legs were too weak to hold me for more than a few minutes at a time, and my left leg was largely paralyzed and seriously atrophied. When I walked, I did so with a cane, and I had a severe rotation forward and to the right. I dragged my left foot and threw it to the side to keep it coming along with me. I usually stayed at Tai Chi class for about a half hour and then went home all pooped out.

My son Sean had told me I really needed to come to Tai Chi class because it would help my balance and improve my energy. If it hadn't been my own son saying I should come, the likelihood of my going to a Tai Chi class would have been about the same as my going to the moon. I didn't know anything about Tai Chi, but I lumped it into the category of all things non-Christian that one such as I would simply have no reason to investigate. I had somewhat similar feelings about it to those I had when I was young toward Pentecostals, or "holy rollers," as we called them then. We didn't know anything about them, but since they were "different," they were suspect and were just as well left alone. The fact that Tai Chi was "eastern" also made it a suspicious activity—it must be somehow connected with eastern religions and mantras and meditation and all of those things that seemed foreign and taboo to good Christians like me.

But Sean was living with us at the time, and I couldn't avoid seeing him doing his Tai Chi workout. The flowing movements were beautiful, peaceful and calming. After he had been doing it for several months, I noticed that it was also having very good effects on his lifestyle. He began hanging out with the Tai Chi crowd, and I discovered that they were a bunch of "clean livers," as we used to call them—no alcohol, no drugs, no caffeine, healthy exercise and good clean fun. Besides that, most of them seemed to be vegetarians. Sean began looking and feeling healthier and gaining an excitement about life that I had not seen him have for a long time. His motivation for work changed dramatically, and he began to apply himself to a new job in computer graphics. Sean was being transformed in front of my eyes in a very positive way, and I saw that it was his Tai Chi connection that was helping him make the change.

Sean started by saying to me, "Mom, you really need to change your diet"—and he handed me the books to help me do so.

Then he began to say, "Mom, this exercise would be really good for you"—and he would show me what to do.

Then it was, "Mom, if you don't do anything else, you really need to breathe, every day"—and he would show me breathing exercises and talk about how it would increase my energy.

At first it was like Sean was speaking to me from a far distant planet. It was hard to hear him, and it was hard to understand why any of it was important or how it could help something as serious as my condition. Nevertheless, he was lovingly there for me.

He came home one night and announced excitedly that he could "feel the chi." I couldn't understand what he was talking about. How could you feel "chi" or "energy?" He showed me how to put my hands close to each other and feel a little "ball" of energy between them. Very strange—but I could feel it! What was this "energy" or "chi?" How could breathing exercises increase *my* energy?

Sean began to tell me about how the "Sifu" would do "bodywork" on his once-broken neck and how the "energy" would then begin to flow to the rest of his body. "What is a Sifu?" I wondered. "Oriental bodywork"—what a strange idea. It sounded like something the Japanese do on their cars after they've been in an accident. What kind of person would do "bodywork?" It sounded so—well—physical!

In January, just as my Jubilee year was getting well underway, Sean invited our youngest son Jeremy to go to Tai Chi class with him. Jeremy, who had burned himself out doing two sports, in addition to maintaining a straight A average in school, was in need of restoration. The "Sifu," who I discovered was also a trainer of professional athletes, offered to work with Jeremy and train him in tennis, as well as in Tai Chi. Who was this "Sifu" anyway, this "Sifu" who does Tai Chi and "bodywork" and trains professional athletes—and now he was offering to train my son?!

I began hearing stories about the Sifu. I heard that he could sense and feel other people's energy. How was that possible? I heard he could direct his own energy to heal people through the bodywork. How could a person "direct" his energy to heal? I heard he was sensitive to other people's thoughts and emotions. I heard he was extremely quick and agile. I heard he looked like he was in his thirties even though he was in his mid-forties. He must be a very interesting fellow.

I first went to Tai Chi class because both Sean and Jeremy were going and because they were experiencing good, healthy results. I continued because, even after a few simple exercises, I began feeling better. This evidence made me willing to explore further. Besides, after one or two classes, I could see that no one was going to proselytize me for Buddhism or Taoism—it was just good, clean exercise!

So there I was on Palm Sunday evening at Ida Noyes Hall on the campus of the University of Chicago. Our church had had a traditional service in the morning, complete with the waving of palms, and I was thinking of the coming Holy Week, of Christ entering into the city in triumph, of Christ fulfilling his destiny by going to the cross, and of Christ rising with victorious power from the grave to open the way to victory for all who came after him. With these thoughts in my mind, I did a few exercises with the Tai Chi class and then walked around in the circle during the break, limping and swinging my leg out as usual.

I had never exchanged more than a few words with the Sifu, who was always engaged in teaching and working with students, and I wasn't sure he really noticed me. On this particular evening, however, as I was limping slowly around, he asked me, "So why are you walking that way, Anna?"

I responded, "Well, I have multiple sclerosis, and my left leg is paralyzed."

He said matter-of-factly, "Nah! It's not paralyzed. Come on over here." He invited me to a corner of the carpeted library in which the class was meeting.

He asked me to lift up my left leg, and I could barely get my foot to come off the floor. "Lie down," he said. It was a surprising instruction, so much so that I did as I was asked.

I lay down on the carpet, and he began to work on my left leg and hip, pressing with his hands and instructing me to "Push, relax, push, relax," while he pressed the leg farther and farther toward my opposite side. It was painful. He did some other manipulations and then said, "Now, get up and walk." I did so. He watched me carefully.

"Okay, lie down again." His strong fingers seemed to penetrate right to the bone of my hip joint, causing me to cry out with pain—but also to feel that something in the joint was moving into proper position.

I got up and walked again, and this time my foot was clearing the floor.

"Lift your leg now," he said.

It came up much higher than before. He looked at me in somewhat the way a sculptor might view the effect of his work and then asked me to lie down so he could work some more.

As he manipulated my muscles, I said, "But my leg is so crooked. It's all turned in."

"Oh, don't worry about that," he said, "I'll take care of that!" and he proceeded to grasp the large muscles of my leg with his penetrating fingers and then twist and mold them around toward their proper alignment, just as a sculptor would manipulate clay. The pain was intense.

After a few moments, he said, "Now get up and try it."

For a moment I felt confused, as though my central processing unit was deleting an old program and loading a new one and the new information was not yet coming up on my screen. I blinked, shook my head and slowly got to my feet. As I did so, I felt a lightness where the old heaviness had been. My leg lifted right up and my foot easily cleared the floor. I brought my thigh parallel with the floor. I looked in astonishment, first at myself and then at him. He looked back matter-of-factly. He said, "Your sciatic nerve was blocked up. I just released it."

My neurologist had been telling me for years that the reason I couldn't walk was because I had a problem with lesions in my brain. This fellow was standing there telling me the problem was in my hip, and he had just proven it beyond question by releasing the hip and helping me walk again—and he had done it in less than twenty minutes!

Later I would discover that Sifu Bruce's simple explanations masked the complex and highly specialized skills he was employing. At that time I just looked at him dumbfounded, trying to assimilate the profusion of thoughts and feelings that came welling up, feelings of amazement, of waving palms and dancing in the streets, of leaping for joy, of triumph and resurrection. They were feelings rising up in a place inside me that is beyond intellect and articulation, an eternal place where actions, events and certainties are already present but not yet manifest, already accomplished but still to be performed, already assured but yet to be experienced, already divinely ordained but requiring human authorization and participation—feelings no words could express.

I looked down at myself and said simply, "I have a lot of work to do."

He nodded. I took his hand, and, feeling that this stranger had just changed my life, I wondered what else I could possibly say. I simply closed my eyes, and from the bottom of my heart I said, "Thank you." He smiled and walked away to work with another person.

That night I went home and began to feel the extraordinary sensations of the nerves in my leg and my whole left side turning on again. I began to have sensations where I had not had any for years—tingling, twitching, latent muscles moving, my foot making little motions up and down. Parts of me that had been dead for years were celebrating their own personal Easter, rising again in joy, saying yes to new life and new possibilities. I rejoiced with them, moving, stretching, celebrating their little victories, praising God for each tiny sign of new life. It was Jubilee, Palm Sunday, and Easter resurrection all rolled into one.

At the same time all the palms were waving, I knew in my heart from the first moment that, indeed, I would have a lot of work to do. Even though that twenty minutes changed my life, I knew that the rest of my healing would not be "instant," that I would not have a divine lightning bolt from on high. Rather, I felt life rising inside me, slowly and surely. I sensed from the beginning that I was intended to experience fully every moment, every feeling, every hope, every disappointment, every frustration, every triumph on my path to healing. I sensed that I was intended to will my healing, participate in it, bring it into full manifestation. I felt that my healing would not be something that was done *to* me but *with* me, that it would be a co-creative adventure in which I would be a full, intentional participant. I sensed a new future opening before me in which I would come to know every nook and cranny of myself in the process of healing, and perhaps I would one day even be able to share it with others. Just as Christ had claimed the his triumph by walking the Via Dolorosa, I would claim mine by walking through my Holy Week of healing, experiencing an unfolding miracle of rising up to new life—all the way to Easter!

Born Again

When a new baby arrives in a household, everything changes. Everyone knows ahead of time, makes plans, re-arranges schedules, creates new expectations and hopes, and prepares to fulfill new roles. Family and friends are notified that a big event will occur, and, when it finally happens, people step in to support the family and share the excitement. It is a joyous time, even though it is full of new challenges for everyone.

My Jubilee Year launched me into a new life as though I were born again. I was "putting off the old" and "putting on the new." I had a new identity, new roles, new healing, new challenges, new hope. I had a new life opening before me, and I felt I was becoming a new person. Unlike the newborn baby, however, no one was expecting my new birth, and no one was prepared ahead of time that it would happen; thus, my arrival on the scene as a new person was a bit shocking to everyone, something like a birth after menopause.

Just like a new child, I needed changes to be made in order to grow and develop—changes in roles, space, schedules, priorities, and support of family and friends. Unfortunately, since mine was not the typical new birth, no one knew what those changes were or how they should happen. Everyone was a little confused. A newborn child is also not aware that she is causing such a big change in the lives of the people around her. She is just learning to breathe, move, see, feel, hear and relate to all the newness around her, discovering how she fits into the whole new scheme of life. In the same way, I was not aware that my "new birth" would shake up the system around me as much as it did. Like a newborn child who has to cry in order make her needs known, I had to become more assertive in order to let people around me know what I needed to live and grow as a new person.

My body was soft and pudgy, and my feet were like baby feet, soft and tender, with no muscles. I hadn't walked for years, so I had to learn to walk all over again. My balance, just like a toddler's, was quite precarious. I wasn't as low to the floor though, so, if I fell down, I had farther to fall and I could injure myself seriously. At first, just getting down the long hallway in our apartment was a challenge. I would hit the wall frequently, usually on the right side, because of my severe rotation to the right.

Every day was a new day with new physical challenges and new attempts to go a little bit farther and do a little more than I did the day before. I would switch back and forth from using the scooter to walking with a cane. Don was like an anxious parent, trying to corral a reckless toddler and prevent injury. I, as the reckless toddler, needed protection, support and encouragement, but I also rebelled against restrictions. I wanted to try everything myself. I wanted to go down the stairs and out the door by myself; I wanted to cross the street and walk down the sidewalk in our residential park; I wanted to take the car and go shopping; I wanted to explore my world—but I didn't know which thing I should do first! Just as a child does not have a sense of which activities are appropriate to a particular stage of development, I did not know which activity or exercise should come next; therefore, I wasn't always able to predict what I could do successfully. When I went too far or did too much, I would exhaust myself, and Don, like the patient parent, would come to the rescue. While I erred on the side of risk, he erred on the side of caution, at first urging me to use my scooter, and, later, to *please* use my cane. I was an adult and too big to order around, but I was also unable to carry out my desired exploits without protection and help. That meant I required time and energy from someone else when everyone's time and energy was already oversubscribed. The result was tension and frustration, with no one knowing what to expect next.

I came to the conclusion that it was much harder to get well than to get sick. When one becomes chronically ill, one just slides down the tube and everyone at the bottom has to grab you as you fall. Things are chaotic for a while, but over time, people's roles become routine and predictable. Family and friends get into a pattern in which they perform their expected functions and also maintain their own lifestyles. When one is getting well, there is a different energy required, an energy of flexibility, adaptation, exploration, uncertainty, of disrupted schedules and expectations.

I was shaking up the system, but I would not be refused. I was no longer dying. I was rising again in new, vigorous birth, growing, changing, becoming a new person with a new life, a new energy, a new will. It was not a blip of momentary change on my progress chart, not a statistical fluctuation, not something operating on me from the outside. I was taking responsibility for my own life and my own health. At the same time, it was not just me—it was God's life in me and my life in God's, and my life together with everyone else's life who was close to me, flowing together in a powerful act of co-creation. We were creating a new person and a new world in which I—and all of us together—could viably, joyously live.

Tai Chi: Exercise I Could Do

After my initial healing on Palm Sunday, I began attending Tai Chi class regularly. The dramatic change in my ability to walk made me want to find out more about this way of treating my disability that was so very different than anything I had known before. It was certainly a major departure from the rehab I had experienced from Western physical therapists! The fact was that one twenty-minute session at Tai Chi class had helped me make more progress than I had made during many sessions of regular physical therapy. I wondered if I could find more of the answers I was looking for.

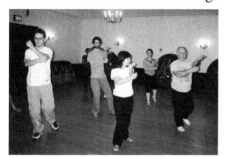

1996: The Tai Chi Class at the University of Chicago.

Sifu Bruce Moran started Tai Chi classes on the University of Chicago campus in 1984, and they met there for 25 years until 2009, led by instructors he trained and certified. Anyone in the University community could attend the classes, and our class at that time included undergraduate and graduate students, faculty members and spouses from physics, biological sciences, law, divinity, business schools and other departments, a medical doctor, and administrative staff. People came to Tai Chi to de-stress from high-powered academics, mid-term all nighters, dissertation pressures, job tensions, and the anxieties of everyday life. Many people came to class because of some health issue, injury or disability that they want to address in a healthy, natural way. Our classes included people with Crohn's disease, asthma, hip and knee injuries, Parkinson's—people with the whole range of human struggles and challenges. And then, of course, there was me. I was the most obviously broken of all.

Sifu Bruce (Sifu is the title of a person who has achieved master status in the art of Tai Chi) did not just "teach a class" but built a unique community of people who shared their skills, their experience and their lives with each other and with whomever came into the class. When I came to class I entered into an open, accepting, non-judgmental environment with caring, compassionate teachers who helped me do what I was able to do without pushing me too far or expecting too much. There was no sense of competition or comparison with anyone else. All students were working on what they needed at their own individual pace. At the same time, there was "good energy"—a sense of camaraderie and shared expectation that we were doing something good for ourselves. I didn't know until years later that these qualities were intentionally built into the class by Sifu Bruce and that they were characteristic of the traditional Taoist healing environment that he had learned from the master teachers before him.

I gradually learned more about Sifu Bruce. He grew up in an Irish/Slovak community in the steel mill area of Chicago's far south side. He comes from hard-working and reflective folks who serve their community and love their country, qualities they passed on to Bruce. He earned an MBA at DePaul University and became politically active. He has continued his political activity over the years, eventually founding Strategic Planning Initiatives, a Chicago/D.C. area consulting and think tank team that works with federal government officials and departments on issues of national concern. For a long time I wondered how the political work fits in with Bruce's commitment to healing and empowering other people to live healthy lives. I learned that it is all part of a desire to serve others.

Sifu Bruce began studying Tai Chi in 1978 at the age of twenty-six and has been teaching for over twenty-five years. He studied under Grand Master Lu Hung-Ping, Sifu John Kotsias, and other well known Tai Chi and martial arts and healing masters from China, Japan, Korea, Okinawa, the Philippines, Thailand, and the United States. This way of preparing for healing is a totally different world than I knew about in the Western system. He has traveled extensively to Asia, studying teachings that have been passed down from teacher to student through the generations.

Bruce speaks with emotion about his teachers and about the history of Tai Chi. The form he teaches is Tai Chi Tao, the Old Yang Tai Chi Classical Family Style in the long form that was practiced by masters in China. He feels it is his responsibility to pass on the purity of this heritage so that it is not shortcut, watered down or commercialized. One of his familiar sayings is, "You can't cheat on the Old Yang Style Family recipe!" The way he teaches his Tai Chi Tao classes incorporates the principles and practices, including healing, that were passed down to him by his master teachers.

Sifu Bruce often expresses his desire to let the blessings of the Creator flow through him. Over a period of twenty-five years he has helped make that happen by putting together a package of healing skills that integrate Tai Chi with Traditional Chinese Medicine, acupuncture and modern Western physical therapy and sports recovery. His specialty is in recovery and rehabilitation of physical and neurological disorders, including formidable diseases like mine, such as MS, Parkinson's and Guillain-Barré Syndrome. He consults, teaches and lectures internationally in Asian medicine, therapeutic recovery and rehabilitation and has developed his own system of recovery, which he calls NAROM (Neurological Adaptive Recovery of Muscles). Bruce has numerous distinguished clients, including Chicago's Mayor Richard Daley and his family.

Sifu Bruce has passed his expertise on through the advanced students he has trained and the teachers he has certified. His students are of greatest importance to him. In his training he wants to preserve the integrity of the Tai Chi Tao art and also respect and honor what students learn in order to develop themselves. Character growth and service to others is an integral part of the training. I observed from my own sons that he was willing to give his time, energy and expertise freely when a person showed the desire to learn, spending many hours in training for which he received no compensation. On the other hand, he would not waste his time on people who were not willing to work. When he took on serious students, he was a rigorous and demanding taskmaster, always challenging their motives and pushing them toward a higher level of performance, physically, mentally and emotionally, in order to bring them up to the high standards his teachers taught him.

The two senior teachers in our class, Sifu Ed Gierut and Mike Farrar, are experienced certified instructors who gently watched over and guided me. Drew Bergerson and Chris Randle are highly trained assistant teachers who began helping me do the Chi Kung and the Old Yang family Style Tai Chi movements. Emil Martinec, a Professor of Physics at the University of Chicago was one of the most seasoned students, practicing and teaching Tai Chi with the same precision he brings to his study of the structural foundations of string theory. Sean, my eldest son, was also assisting in the class. As I continued with classes three times a week, I discovered that I was surrounded by people whose kindness, warmth and generosity would not only lay the groundwork for my future healing but would also become friends and companions on my life journey

Martial demos were somewhat rare at class because Sifu Bruce emphasizes Tai Chi for its benefits of health and healing and reserves

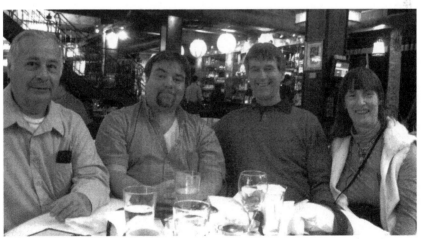

2008: Anna and her Tai Chi teachers, Sifu Ed Gierut, Certified Instructor Michael Farrar, and Sifu Bruce Moran.

martial training for advanced students. I noticed right away that Bruce would circulate around among students, checking in with them and talking softly about how they were doing. Sometimes he would surprise a student by telling one of his signature jokes. Often he would call a person to the side and do some manipulation to relieve stress or injury. Sean benefited from this skill when Sifu restored much of the range of motion that was lost in his neck when it was broken years before. I knew the distress Sean had endured because of his neck, and I was amazed that it could be relieved with no surgery through skillful bodywork. I observed that the healing Sean and I experienced was not something unusual—it was an integral part of the class. While bodywork is unusual and the results may seem extraordinary to us Westerners, it is a skill that is well known in China and other Eastern countries.

Sifu Bruce regularly held little lectures during class in which he talked about principles of Tai Chi and how to achieve better overall health. He covered breathing, self massage and acupressure, nutrition and even protection from cold during the blustery Chicago winters. Sometimes he would do a full-fledged lecture on various aspects of Tai Chi Tao and related arts.

Disabled—and Doing Tai Chi!

I was an unusual participant in the Tai Chi class. Other students couldn't help but wonder about me as I tottered around unsteadily on my feet, sat down to rest for a while, attempted a few Chi Kung moves and then left after a short time exhausted. Flora, who was then the Director of Women's Studies at Northwestern University Hospital, is one person who had a strong emotional response. She told me later that she was actually angry that my family was bringing me to Tai Chi class and raising my hopes that something could be done for my condition: "It was so obvious just from looking at you that your situation was beyond help." Then she looked at me with raised eyebrows and pursed lips and said, "How wrong I was!" I went to class regardless of how hopeless I looked to others, and I found there were things I could do from the very beginning that helped me begin my recovery.

Warm Ups. The warm-ups that always came at the beginning of the two-hour class were designed by Sifu Bruce to gently bring the body up to a basic, functional level of movement. They consist of a variety of circular, elliptical, and spiral motions that limber up the muscles and lubricate the joints so they move smoothly and synergistically, allowing the free coursing of internal energy or "chi" through the body. The movements are simple and yet powerful. As I repeated them over and over again, week after week, they began turning on and tuning up my frazzled nervous system. I developed more muscle tone and coordination and felt a new energy I had not known for many years. It was a psychological boost to do the exercises with a whole crowd of healthy college students who were taking them just as seriously as I was!

Warm-ups usually started with putting the feet parallel and shifting the weight from side to side, smoothly and evenly; then moving one foot forward at a forty-five degree angle and shifting the weight; then doing various weight shifting patterns on both sides. The weight-shifting exercises were very basic but important for learning the progressively more difficult moves. They were vital for me because I didn't know how to shift my weight—I had to learn the most fundamental movements all over again. Gentle, repeated motions began developing some muscle tone in my legs and hips.

Stepping exercises involved stepping and shifting the weight on the balls of the feet in an X pattern on the floor. Doing these stepping patterns over and over began to neurologically re-train me so that I could step in various directions with more control and confidence. I didn't know at the time that the warm-ups and "universal stepping exercises" were unique to our group, a product of Bruce Moran's genius in biomechanics.

The warm-up moves were all preparatory for "Chi Kung," which was nearly always the second part of the class. Chi Kung is a series of slow, deliberate movements that are designed to increase and balance the flow of "chi" or energy through the body. There is very specific training in how to place the feet, move each part of the body, shift weight, and exercise balance and coordination, all while breathing and maintaining focus. Chi Kung opens up the "micro-cosmic orbit" so that energy begins to flow through the body's two major "meridians" – called the Governing (Yang) Meridian and the Conceptual (Yin) Meridian. The terms and concepts were all strange, but it seemed similar to learning a foreign language—except that this language also employed body language as an integral part of its meaning. It was the whole body speaking, not just the mind and tongue.

Chi Kung. There are many varieties of Chi Kung, but the one we beginners did most often is a basic set of eight movements taught to Sifu Bruce by his teacher, Sifu John Kotsias, the author of *The Essential Movements of Tai Chi*. This set can take up to an hour, but at first I just did what I was able to do. The first movement is a standing posture called "Heaven," and it involves standing still with feet together. This seemingly simple posture was very difficult for me. The instructions were issued in a calm, rhythmic way:

> "Feet together, knees slightly bent, back straight, as though suspended from a string through the top of the head. Shoulders down, hips tucked, tongue lightly touching the roof of the mouth. Breathe from the diaphragm. Do the microcosmic orbit, collecting the energy in the dan tien (a place below and behind the navel), then circulating it from the dan tien, down between the legs, up the spine and neck, over the top of the head, down the center of the front and then to the dan tien once again."

The next posture, called "holding the ball," also appeared simple enough, but it was even more difficult for me than the first. It involved getting into a "horse" type of stance with the feet a shoulder's width apart and the knees out. The arms are held in somewhat of a circular shape at about shoulder level. Subsequent moves become progressively more difficult in terms of balance and coordination.

The instructors would demonstrate and explain the proper postures and movements and how they promote balance and coordination, strength, endurance, and development of the body's internal energy. Then they would go around correcting each student's posture. I had very little sense of myself and my physical alignment, so these corrections were very important in helping me become aware of how I was handling my body. Watching other people intentionally modeling what was healthy and correct gave me a vision of what I needed to do for myself. The instructions for the moves became a part of my internal CD collection that I played over and over to myself while I worked on each posture. Sean and Jeremy gave me pointers and encouragement at home.

When Sean said, "Mom, if you don't do anything else, you have to breathe," I wondered what planet he came from. I thought, "Isn't that what everyone on Earth does all the time, if they're alive? What does breathing have to do with improving my health?" I certainly had no intention to stop breathing! As I attended class, I gradually started to understand the importance of breathing in a rhythmic, intentional way from the lower and middle diaphragm. Each of the Tai Chi moves is accompanied by coordinated breathing. Inhaling (yin) is for contracting movements and drawing in energy. Exhaling (yang) is for expanding movements and extending energy.

We often did a series of breathing exercises in class, accompanied by movements designed to help energy flow through the "meridians." I didn't know what "meridians" were, but I certainly felt the benefits when I followed the instructions. Intentional breathing accompanied every exercise, helping me to loosen and relax the muscles and joints more effectively. Breathing also supported my concentration, giving me a focal point for my attention as I worked through the exercises. The breathing and exercise was invigorating. Even if I came to class tired, I always left feeling relaxed, refreshed, and energized. More advanced students took the breathing to a higher level to increase the flow of chi and create a more dynamic mind and body dialogue.

Eventually the breathing helped me build my energy so that it dispersed the terrible coldness in my body. For about fifteen years I had been extremely sensitive to cold and had been unable to control my body temperature. This is typical of people who have MS. Going out on a frigid Chicago day would turn my feet into icy blocks that took a long time to thaw with heating pads or soaking in a hot tub. How many nights I recall being unable to sleep because of numbing cold in my extremities! Breathing gave me a way of warming myself up. I would start to build the energy and warmth by breathing and focusing on the *dan tien,* the point two-and-a-half to three inches below and behind my navel. This point is also called the "cauldron" or "lower burner"—and I found out why. Building up the energy there by breathing is like firing up a furnace. Once this area was good and hot, I would start the heat moving by visualizing it going out to my extremities to warm up my cold hands and feet. It was much more effective than a hot water bottle or heating pad, and I carried the heat source of my breath with me at all times! I did not know until later that the breathing was also helping me fight viruses and Candida yeast by oxygenating my body, increasing my pH levels, and stimulating the peristaltic action of my intestinal tract. I was discovering that breath is life. A whole new dimension of meaning was opening to me as I understood why "breath" is also theologically associated with "spirit," which is the active, creative, life-giving agent throughout all creation. Breath was giving me new life, energy and spirit.

Tai Chi Form. The practice of Chi Kung prepares one for learning the Tai Chi form, which is a series of flowing, harmonious movements involving the whole body. There are three "parts" to the Old Yang Family Classical Tai Chi form, with the first and simplest taking most people up to a year to learn and the second and third parts taking four or five years to complete. Many students came to class and proceeded through the first and second parts while I struggled along for about four years to learn the first part. There are still sections of it

I don't do well because of the lack of muscular strength in my lower left side. Nevertheless, I can still say, having started out not even being able to walk, that I am the "Most Improved Player!"

Learning the Chi Kung and Old Yang Family Style Tai Chi form helped me locate myself in space and learn to move in three dimensions. I had been sitting and looking straight ahead for several years, and when I moved I was jerky and unbalanced, especially when turning corners and changing direction. The form required that I learn to move around, exercising the muscles to shift, turn, step, bend, squat, push and do other movements in a smooth, controlled fashion. Doing the movements over and over began to re-train me physically and neurologically. I began to sense and feel and control my body, and it began to do what I wanted instead of whatever it randomly decided to do on its own.

Sensitivity Training. At first, I had no idea what sensitivity training was. If someone had asked me, I suppose I would have thought of people sitting around in a circle pressing hands and sending telepathic messages around to each other. As it happened, we did several sessions of sensitivity training before someone told me what we were doing. It wasn't anything like what I had thought. We would begin in a standing posture, tightening and releasing the right foot and ankle, then the right knee, then the right hip, right waist, right shoulder and neck, right side of the face and head, and then finally the entire right side. Then we would proceed likewise up the left side and finish by tightening and loosening the entire body. The intentional tightening and loosening of specific muscles in sequence, helped me become "sensitive" to my muscles and how they were or were not functioning—and that was "sensitivity training." As I became aware of my various muscles and how they feel when they are working and not working, I gained increasing control over their function and was able to address my body's specific needs. I would note where I was tight or numb or in pain and intentionally relax or send energy to the needed place in my body.

Energy Bodywork. Coming from a conservative, Christian, Midwestern background, I had a tendency to associate massage with steamy, storefront tattoo parlors on little back streets where prostitutes and druggies hang out. Either that, or with luxurious clubs where gorgeous, muscular blondes work on mafia men or James-Bond-type hunks. Besides that, massage just seemed too "physical" for ethereal, spiritual types like me. Well, what we did in Tai Chi class didn't fit any of those ideas—there was nothing steamy or James Bondy at all. Students would pair up and follow the examples and explanations of the teachers as they demonstrated various techniques in a standing posture. I didn't know the name of it at the time, but what we did was not really massage—it was Taoist energetic bodywork, incorporating elements of Tuina, Shiatsu, and Nuad Boran (Chinese, Shiatsu and Thai bodywork), acupressure, and meridian healing therapy based on Traditional Chinese Medicine (TCM). Sifu Bruce and the other instructors modeled and instructed us as we pressed points down the sides of the spine, down and up, and then farther away from the spine, down and up. Then we would do the three-pronged pressure points at the shoulders, learning several techniques for relieving stress and tension there. Then we would move down the upper arms, then the forearms and then to the hands—ah! hand massage, how wonderful! At the end we would "tap out" by cupping the palms and vigorously slapping the back, followed by "brushing out" down the shoulders, off the arms and hands and then down to the feet, providing a lovely sense of refreshment and relaxation.

The energy bodywork became a powerful healing tool. It helped me discover where my major muscle groups are and which places are likely to hold tension. I learned that tension is manifest in hard, lumpy, knotty muscles and that I had a lot of muscles that fit that description. I was a "knotty girl" even if I was not a "naughty" one. As we practiced bodywork, Sifu Bruce would explain how we were manipulating and utilizing the acupressure points in the body to achieve certain effects. Working points around the shoulders and neck could disperse symptoms of colds and flu. Sometimes pressing a point in one part of the body would affect function in a part farther away. For example, rubbing a certain spot on the feet could have the effect of clearing the lungs! I also learned that bodywork stimulates the internal organs, bringing the whole body system into better function. All of this helped me think of my body as a unified system rather than as parts that work separately. As we learned how to manipulate many acupressure points during bodywork, I felt the benefits of relaxation, improved movement, and energy.

Practicing bodywork on other people helped build my awareness and skill so that I could work on myself. I began working on my knots at home, and Sean and Jeremy also helped me out by massaging my sore, aching muscles. As the knots and "hot spots" relaxed, I was able to feel warm energy flowing into the surrounding tissues, bringing my dormant body to life. Sometimes I could feel energy begin to flow through my whole body, improving my ability to sense, feel and move. While there is no doubt that I had neurological damage from the multiple sclerosis, I learned by practicing bodywork that a significant part of my immobility was due to tense, tight muscles and to those tight muscles impinging on nerve pathways. I needed to enhance nerve function in any way I could and found I could do that to a surprising extent by straightening my body, removing the blockages and loosening the muscles through which the nerves had to pass. All of these insights came through personal experience. It would be much later that I would discover the research describing the benefits more scientifically.

The most important thing about Tai Chi for me was that it offered something I could do from the very beginning and that I could continue to build for many years to come as I became stronger and more independent. The more I practiced Tai Chi, the more I developed a sense that the body has its own integrity and that it "speaks" powerfully about how it feels and what it needs. Tai Chi was teaching me the language of my body. As I learned it, I felt less and less that my disease was a set of symptoms that was victimizing me. I began to feel a sense of wholeness and unity, a sense of self control, a sense of becoming a whole person who is able to understand what is good for me, make my own decisions, and direct my actions in ways that are good for me.

Yes, it's true that Tai Chi and Sifu Bruce's approach to healing are strange to people from my background, but his methods are natural and effective, and at heart he has values that are similar to mine. I began to see that his spiritual life is as important to him as mine and that his desire to let the blessings of the Creator flow in him is rooted in the love of God. At the core he is moved by compassion—or he wouldn't bother with the likes of me! I began to speak the language of "blessing" to him and to everyone in the Tai Chi class, viewing them all as part of God's gift of life to me. I felt that God had led me to Tai Chi and that in some way I did not understand Bruce was providing the answers to the prayers for healing that hundreds of people had been praying for me for many years. I still had questions, but I had enough evidence of God at work that I was willing to hold them in my heart, expecting that I would come to understanding in due time.

I joyously shared my experiences of healing with family and friends and also gave testimonies at church about what was happening, praising God for each new advance. I had a happy naiveté that everyone would be as thrilled about my progress as I was. After all, they had been praying earnestly for my healing for years! Probably they would have been more comfortable if my healing had come through a more traditional source, such as medication, physical therapy or—best of all, of course—a straight-down, bona fide, certified, walking-and-leaping miracle at the church altar. When I related a new skill and described how Bruce helped me achieve it, I began to see smiles fade. My friends did not understand what was happening to me or how it was happening. "So who *is* this 'Sifu,' and what is he doing with Anna? Is this an appropriate activity for a Baptist minister?" My practice of Tai Chi was beginning to raise questions among my friends.

Easternizing My Healing

In the fall of 1996, a series of events occurred that shook my faith in Western approaches to physical rehabilitation—at least for my particular problems. I did not have a successful experience with traditional physical therapy through our local hospital. One young female therapist threw her hands up in frustration and exclaimed, "You have so many asymmetries! Do you realize that you're a prime candidate for hip and joint replacement if you keep walking that way?" —as though threats and prophecies of doom would get me to straighten up more quickly!

Just because the University of Chicago Hospital was a prestigious institution didn't mean it had all the solutions for people with severe problems such as mine. Only one therapist at that time had some skill in working with neurological disorders. Myra was a young Irish woman with genuine compassion and skill. She worked my arms and legs and did electrical nerve stimulation that gradually helped turn some of my nervous system back on and stimulated some of my atrophied muscles to start firing again. She regularly strapped me into a complicated machine that exercised my ankle flexors. It had a little screen that I could watch to see how much pressure I was exerting in pulling up my foot, the usual reading being about zero for me because I had no strength in my left ankle. It was hard work, and after each session I was tired. She gave me exercises to do, and I did them at home. Nevertheless, progress was slow and painful.

It was on a Wednesday that Myra fitted me with a simple, flexible brace for my left foot that would keep it from dropping and help it swing through to create a smoother gait. On that day she also put me on the electronic machine that exercised my foot and measured the strength of the upward pull, which, as usual, registered at about zero.

The following day, Thursday, I went to Tai Chi class and Sifu observed that I had the brace on. He told me that wearing a brace would inhibit my exercising the foot so that it could return to normal. He emphasized the natural healing capacity of the body and said that my foot needed to be neurologically re-trained as well as physically strengthened. I took the brace off and pointed at the foot, which was hanging there limply, and said, "Can you do anything about that?"

He looked at the foot, thought a moment and said, "Yes, I can do that." Then, to my astonishment, he began to work on my head, not my foot. He did some gentle touching, saying, "Okay, it's blocked up there and there." He has the ability to sense and feel the flow of energy through people's bodies and uses words like "blocked up" to accommodate those who are not familiar with physiological terminology. Then he began to do some penetrating work on "knots" that were in various parts of my temples and the back portion of my head. It was painful, but as the knots released I began to feel warmth flowing down through my neck and spine and to my lower body. All of a sudden I was able to pull my foot up! Up and down, up and down—something I hadn't been able to do for years! The ankle was very weak and I could only do a few repetitions, but it was a start. Sifu described what he did as "cranial-sacral therapy," "neurological point release," and "fascial release."

The next day I went back to see Myra and came walking in without the brace. She saw me coming from a distance and said happily, "Wow, the brace is really helping you! You're walking so much better!"

Smiling, I said, "Well, actually I'm not wearing the brace."

"You're not?" she asked in amazement. "What happened?"

I told her the story of the previous evening as she listened with wide eyes and a slight jaw drop.

"Well," she said, "I had some training in that, but I never saw anyone get any results with it. I'll tell you what. Let's go put you on the machine and get a reading on your ankle flexion today."

That was an exciting idea, because it would be a comparison of my performance immediately before the cranial sacral work and immediately afterward. She strapped me into the machine and we watched as the reading went way up above ten, at least ten points higher than I had ever achieved before.

Myra was stunned. "I can't believe it," she said. "I have to share this at our staff meeting." She asked if I thought Bruce would be able to come and demonstrate his work to other therapists. I collected Sifu's credentials and gave them to her, but she was not able to generate enough interest among the staff to bring him in for a session. Bruce was not surprised. The skills he has are not well understood in the West and are not in the mainstream of traditional Western practice, even though they are well known and practiced in the Orient. Thus, what he does is not recognized as being a legitimate approach to therapy, and response by traditional practitioners is a blend of skepticism, disdain and indifference. Even though we had documented the benefits of the cranial-sacral work on me, my example was treated as "anecdotal" and thus as having little importance. I knew that science does not function on "anecdotal" evidence, but my need for help was not going to wait around for a couple of generations while a new scientific paradigm was being developed and therapists were trained in new techniques. I wanted to go for the gold now.

The whole experience was a big step toward my disillusionment with traditional rehabilitation programs as being able to address my personal physical and neurological problems. I decided I would just have to consider myself as one piece of anecdotal evidence that could potentially come together with a lot of other people's anecdotal evidence and eventually call the old system into question, challenging it to change. Before long, Myra had to go back to Ireland to help her sick mother, and I was left floating around among therapists who had no idea what to do with me. After a while I abandoned the whole traditional rehabilitation system and concentrated on Tai Chi, because it was helping me much more effectively than anything else.

I continued to go to Tai Chi class, where Sifu Bruce regularly did bodywork for me. The rebuilding of my body was a gradual process. He used a variety of oriental bodyworking techniques, including Thai, Chinese, and Japanese, blended together with protocols he developed from his years of practice. He brought modern therapeutic practice

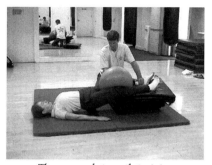
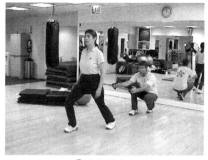

Therapy and strength training with Bruce Moran. *Gait training.*

together with Eastern approaches to create powerful, effective, innovative modes of healing. He would do some straightening and then give me exercises to strengthen and habituate the new alignment into my daily activities. Each small change caused a corresponding change of the muscular structure throughout my body as I rebalanced and reoriented my posture. Since I was in class three times a week, Sifu had opportunity to observe me carefully and judge when I was ready for another adjustment. Frequently the adjustments would take only five minutes or so, but sometimes they took considerably longer. He always knew exactly what I needed and was able to recommend exercises that would support the follow-up. I would leave class feeling energized and empowered to continue my rehab.

Having had several therapists who were clueless about how to help me, I came to appreciate Bruce's skill. Eventually, by mutual agreement, he took charge of my whole healing program, including diet, exercise, bodywork, herbal therapy and recommendations for such procedures as acupuncture and chiropractic work. I began to have two-hour professional sessions with him every four to six weeks. My healing was taking on a strong Eastern flavor.

A Grace Place Healing

The more I practiced Tai Chi and meditation, the more I developed the ability to sense and feel "chi." I could feel the energy flowing in my body and sense it with my hands. Sean and Jeremy and I learned from working with Bruce that the "chi" could be focused and directed to produce healing for oneself or for other people. We wanted to explore how this happens, and I wanted to relate it to my understanding and experience of healing in Christianity. We began to "experiment" on each other, sensing and feeling the energy as we applied massage and also by moving the hands slightly off the body. I was a good candidate for the experiments because there was always plenty wrong with me. I was like a self-contained healing laboratory! Jeremy and I even went to a full-day workshop on therapeutic touch, led by a woman who teaches it to nurses in area hospitals.

One evening I was preparing to go out to a meeting when I rounded a corner in the workout room and my wayward left foot flew out and hit a sharp metal object on the floor. The blow created a nasty puncture on the top of my foot, which quickly began to swell into a bruise. I yelled in pain and sat in a heap on the floor, nursing the foot. I rubbed it tearfully, thinking that now I wouldn't be able to go out and would probably have a sore foot for days.

Sean heard my cry and came to my rescue. Very lovingly, he sat me in a chair and then quietly knelt at my feet and placed his hands on the injury. As he wrapped his hands around the foot and began to lightly stroke it, I could feel heat from his hands begin to penetrate, relieving the pain. He focused intently, breathing quietly and gently, and I could sense his love for me. After about five minutes, my foot was free of pain, and there was a delicious warmth flowing through it. I looked down and saw the swelling had subsided. Even the gash was closed up. I tested the foot and it felt good! I gave Sean a loving hug and went out to my meeting. I had just had my first healing from Sean.

On February 12, 1997, less than a month after my ordination in January, I was experiencing a lot of pain in my back. I had also been having more than the usual number of "explosions" of heat in my body. These explosions, which are experienced by many people with MS, occurred especially when I was under stress and always left me weak and feeling like I had frayed wires running all through my body. Explosions of heat would often alternate, especially at night, with feelings of numbing cold. I was nursing my painful back when Jeremy went by and saw my distress. He asked me to lie down, and he put his hands on my back. It felt like I was getting a deep, penetrating heat treatment. As he focused his energy, the heat went deep into the muscles and then, it seemed, right into my kidneys and other organs. All the tension went out of my back. Then, slowly, he did the same on my left hip, my leg, and then my foot, sensing and focusing energy either with his hands on my body or somewhat off of it. Before long he said, "Oh, Mom, there's something very cold." He began to earnestly focus and to move his hands as though he were pushing something up and away, up and away, in vigorous, waving motions. Then he moved his hands off the body in slow, gentle, soothing motions. When he finished, I felt much better.

I sat up, and we sat there on the floor together. I said, "What did you feel, Jeremy?"

He said solemnly, "It was so cold, Mom."

"What do you think it was, Love?"

He paused a moment and said quietly, "It was the MS ghost." He dropped his eyes. Another pause. He looked at me softly and said, "But I didn't get it all out, Mom."

"The MS ghost?" I silently pondered what he meant, then said, "What do you mean you couldn't you get it out, Jeremy?"

"I didn't have enough faith, Mom," he said seriously.

Jeremy was only seventeen at the time, but he sounded old and wise. I felt God's spirit was giving him deep insight far beyond his years. I pondered what he meant by "the MS ghost." He was selecting language by intuition for an experience that was beyond his normal vocabulary. It seemed that he could sense and feel what was happening, but he did not have the maturity, experience and "faith" to conclude the task of "getting it out," whatever "it" was.

That was on a Wednesday. The following day I was experiencing a lot of stress from a very difficult case of ministry, a woman with multiple personalities and extremely complex family issues. I usually had my guard up when dealing with her, but on this day my defenses were low. Her foul spirit came flashing toward me, sizzling the phone wires and darting right into my heart like lightning. My nervous system exploded with heat, and I put down the phone, feeling seared, weak and disoriented.

That night I went to Tai Chi class barely able to walk and feeling very disconnected emotionally and psychologically. All of our Thursday classes took place at Grace Episcopal Church, commonly known as "Grace Place," in the South Loop. Founded in 1851, Grace Church is the second oldest church in Chicago, an institution of God's blessing for over 150 years. The class that night was occurring in the main sanctuary on the second floor, a setting we used on some rare occasions. The sanctuary has movable furniture and was made available for our use by the Rector, Reverend Ted Curtis, who was a long-time member of our class. Our movements were quiet and meditative, and all of us felt that a church sanctuary was an appropriate place for Tai Chi. Being there in that place, surrounding the central altar, we felt a special sense of peace at the same time our bodies were being refreshed in movements that were a kind of "body prayer." It was a lovely setting for an experience of life and rejuvenation. Later I would realize that this sanctuary was God's special gift, prepared by the prayers and praises of many people over many years for the event that would occur that night. At the time I was not consciously aware of any of that. I was too caught up in my own trouble.

The distress I was feeling that night was apparent to Sifu Bruce, Sifu Ed Gierut, and assistant instructor Chris Randle. As Sifu Bruce was moving around among the various students, he came to me and said, "So, what's going on with you?" I was not able to give a coherent answer. He said, compassionately but matter-of-factly, "Don't worry, I'll get it out. You'll be okay." Once again the words "it" and "get it out" were used, but I was too confused to think about it.

In the sanctuary of Grace Place there is a dividing wall between the sanctuary and the space surrounding it, and the dividing wall has large, arch-shaped openings all the way around. Sifu and I went behind the dividing wall, and he laid down a mat for bodywork, as he had many times before. The Tai Chi class was continuing just through an opening inside the sanctuary. I lay down on the mat, and he began to work, kneeling on the floor next to me. He began working on my solar plexus area with total calm and assurance, penetrating with his strong fingers, deep into my abdomen. It was extremely painful, and I responded at various times with yelling, groaning, coughing and heaving. Those who were in the Tai Chi class that night said they would never forget it because they could hear my cries and sense how much pain I was in. Their quiet, calm movements, which continued throughout this time, were like a prayer, sustaining the profound work that was going on inside me. Bruce must have worked on me for at least a half hour. Then he sat and talked to me and offered me Kleenex as a flood of emotion poured out. As the tears rolled, my body began to relax, and I felt like a huge weight was lifted. When I was quiet, he did some work on my legs to help me walk straight again, and then I just sat there and rested. When the others were taking a break, he told them to keep clear of the area where I was sitting. That night I went home feeling warm and peaceful.

The next day was Valentine's Day, 1997. As I pondered the events of the previous evening, I tried to find some way of thinking about what had happened to me. I recalled the stories in scripture where Jesus freed people from spirits or demons. I wondered if I had been "exorcised." I wondered if that's what Jeremy had meant by describing what he was feeling as "the MS ghost." I recalled times when I had prayed for people to be delivered from spiritual oppression, and they had behaved in similar ways to what I experienced the night before.

In the meantime, it seemed I had a battle on my hands to hold the ground I had gained. That night Sean and Jeremy were in the living room talking until very late. I went to bed feeling warm, but shortly after midnight I felt a terrible coldness trying to take hold of me. It seemed to be coming from outside of me, and as it came I was gripped by horrible fear. I prayed with all the energy I could pray, but it seemed like it was stronger than I was. I knew I needed to breathe to warm myself up and that I needed to circulate warm energy through my body, but I was unable to do so—the cold was overwhelming me, an icy presence enveloping my entire body. I shivered in bed and finally swung my feet to the floor and wrapped a wool blanket around me. My hands and feet felt deathly cold. I put my feet in warm slippers and traversed the long hall to the living room where Sean and Jeremy were quietly talking. I told them I needed their help and their prayers.

I lay down and they began to focus, sensing and feeling with their hands somewhat off my body as they prayed. They both sensed something very cold, and, intuitively, they began moving their hands in motions to send the coldness up and away. After a while I began to feel warm, and they both agreed that the coldness was gone. We sat together until I felt quiet and peaceful.

Those healing experiences at Grace Place and at my home that week in 1997, were God's valentine to me. Since that time, I have never had the same kind of coldness, nor have I had the terrible explosions of unnatural heat. As a matter of fact, it was at about that time that my autonomic nervous system turned back on and I was once again able to perspire and experience normal thermal functioning. For years I had been extremely sensitive to heat and cold and could not tolerate hot weather because I could not perspire. Soon I was able to function normally in hot weather and was able to exercise more because I could release the body heat I generated through perspiration.

It was a landmark experience that changed my life forever. Even so, it was a work of Grace so deep and so profound that I could not talk about it for many years. Like many acts of pure Grace, the surpassing, boundless magnanimity of it broke out of the finitude of time, space, doctrine, and imagination, transcending my capacity for understanding and expression. The process of healing was so intense that I could not deal with everything at once. It would take me years to come to terms with what happened to me at Grace Place. I hid it in my heart for a later time.

Food for Life

My food changes disturbed the Universe even more than my newfound energy and my practice of Tai Chi. Sean brought me *The Multiple Sclerosis Diet Book* by Roy Laver Swank and Barbara Brewer Dugan, and I was so impressed with the research that I immediately changed my diet to meet Swank's recommendations.

Some of the Swank diet instructions include:
- No red meat for the first year, including dark meat of chicken and turkey
- Only 3 ounces of red meat once a week after the first year.
- Eliminate dairy products containing 1 percent butterfat or more except for one serving with 1 gram of butterfat once a day.
- No processed foods with saturated fat.
- Saturated fat cannot exceed 15 grams per day
- Unsaturated fat should be a minimum of 20 grams per day and a maximum of 50 grams per day.

The Swank diet introduced plenty of frustration within our household. My husband was a "meat and potatoes" man and loved his red meat. He was the one fixing a large percentage of the main meals, because I was still not strong enough to do so. He also did all of the shopping. In order to keep the food budget down when all the boys were home, Don had a habit of making a monthly shopping excursion to various food outlets and warehouse-type stores. He would push two carts and have one of the boys push another. Then, being quite familiar with our particular foods, he would head down the aisles, hardly even looking at the shelves, and heave enormous quantities of food into the baskets. He never read labels, partly because he didn't know how and didn't want to take the time and partly because he had vision problems and couldn't read the fine print without stopping, putting his glasses on, and looking very carefully. When he was finished shopping, he would bag it all up, bring it home and lasso any able bodies he could find to help him store it into our large pantries, freezers and refrigerators. He would not expect to go to the store again for a month except for milk and eggs. About every three months I would call a wholesale meat company and order a quarter of beef, some turkeys and various other frozen meats and vegetables, and they would deliver it and put it in the basement freezer.

My new food needs threw Don into confusion. Now he wasn't sure what to get or what to fix. While many of his recipes contained chicken and turkey, many also contained red meat. He had so many responsibilities in taking care of his career and the family that he didn't want to think about what he was doing in the store or the kitchen. He was a big guy, and it was a big kitchen, and he moved fast. He just wanted everyone to clear the path so he could go on automatic pilot and get the job done. Now I was not only changing his habits because of my new mobility, I was also tinkering with the family food chain.

Food changes, especially in a large, complex household, do not come easily. I began accompanying Don on some shopping trips, going down the aisles on my scooter, reading labels and selecting items that were suitable for me. The requirement for low fat required a different cooking style, and changing from saturated oils to olive oil also created added expense. Before long I began making my own meal alongside the meal everyone else was eating—so we had two meals going. Don felt somewhat hurt that his cooking wasn't "good enough" for me and didn't understand what all the diet fuss was about. He had become the Director of the Sloan Digital Sky Survey, a new, high-tech telescope designed to map the universe, and issues surrounding its finances and management were highly contentious. My healing was creating added stress for him at a time when he was experiencing the greatest career challenges of his life. Unfortunately, I knew my healing couldn't wait for his life to become "normal"—we didn't even know what "normal" was! I thought maybe some of my new insights could help him with challenges he was facing, but he had no time to think about it. Even when overweight, high blood pressure and diabetes were taking their toll, he couldn't slow down. I went forward with my diet on my own, and the results for my health were good. I followed the Swank diet instructions for a full year before implementing further changes in my diet. My energy, health and mobility improved.

No dairy. During the initial year I was on the Swank diet, I was getting a great deal of information and encouragement from Sifu Bruce and from the people in our Tai Chi group regarding diet. We would eat together two or three times a week, with Bruce doing the ordering, and we would discuss all kinds of issues related to diet. Sifu, raised in an Irish/Slovak neighborhood on Chicago's Southside, is a reformed meat eater who can describe in detail the effect of a great variety of foods on the body. Several people in the group had special health or dietary needs, and they were also able to share the benefits or drawbacks of different foods in relation to their conditions. One person had overcome extremely severe asthma through diet, acupuncture, yoga and Tai Chi. Others were successfully fighting Herpes virus, colonitis, lactose intolerance, panic attacks, TMJ, endometriosis, malaria and arthritis. Most people in the group were some shade of vegetarian or vegan (no animal products). At that time, vegetarians were even fewer then than they are now (currently somewhere around 2% of the population). I had never really been around any vegetarians before, so it was all a new experience.

Initially I wondered if anyone could even survive without eating meat. Where would they get their protein! Then there were the vegans—strange creatures indeed! There is a star named Vega, and I had recently seen a sci-fi movie in which creatures from that star system were called "Vegans." I thought the earthly variety was just about as strange as those aliens from another star system. Why would anyone want to eat that way? I thought of hippies, tree huggers, environmentalists and animal rights activists, all of whom were way out on the fringe, as far as I was concerned. Nevertheless, I began paying careful attention to the conversations, and I learned that dairy products could be exacerbating some of my MS symptoms, especially the joint and muscle pain. After a year of being on limited dairy, I went all the way to vegan (with the exception of eggs) in the summer of 1997. No animal products! Don looked at me like I had landed from Vega.

Going Organic. Dr. John R. Lee's book, *What Your Doctor May Not Tell You About Menopause* offered me some new insights into the serious disruption of my normal menstruation throughout many years of MS. Dr. Lee provides a well-researched, in-depth discussion of "xenobiotics" or "xenoestrogens," which are foreign substances originating outside the body that cause hormone-like and estrogen-like activity in the body, and thus have a profound impact on hormone balance. He notes that nearly all xenobiotics are petrochemically based (derived from petroleum oil) and describes their pervasive distribution in our environment and in our food supply. They are in the pesticides used to grow our food, in the meat we eat, especially in red meat and dairy fats, in fish through pollution of water, in plastics, cosmetics, toiletries, household cleaners and sprays, detergents, dish soaps, diaphragm gels, spermicides, gels on condoms—and a huge variety of other places and products. He describes us as living in a "sea of estrogens" that can contribute to reproductive abnormalities, cancer, including increasing numbers of cancers of the reproductive tract, infertility, low sperm counts, and the feminization of males.

I knew that MS attacks often occur when the immune system is triggered in some way, and Dr. Lee's book raised my awareness that the environment is full of toxins that could be triggering my immune system. He suggests eating organic foods as one way of reducing intake of these toxins and also encourages discontinuing use of personal and household products containing petrochemicals. I discovered that my Tai Chi friends had already incorporated organic eating into their lifestyles and that several of them belonged to a sustainable fresh-produce coop. They were not only vegetarians but also, as I might have suspected, tree huggers and environmentalists too! During our mealtimes we discussed what products could be substituted for those with the petrochemicals.

Then, once again, a family member stepped in with encouragement to make the personal step into territory I would not otherwise have dared. Chandler, our third son, was running the summer marketing program for a sustainable organic agriculture project near Oberlin College. He was a hands-on advocate of all aspects of environmental protection and organic nutrition, not just for human health but also for the health of the planet. He added his voice to the others, and I was convinced. I decided to take the next step and clean up my life by going natural and organic. I was quickly becoming one of *them*!

It was bad enough when I didn't eat red meat, but, when I went off all meat and all dairy and also wanted to go organic, "all hell broke loose" in the family food arena. By that time Don and I were the only ones left at home, because Maurice was at Bard, Chandler was at Oberlin, and Jeremy, our youngest, had just gone to the University of Florida. Our oldest son Sean had moved out on his own to another Chicago neighborhood. Even though there was less cooking to do, the entire food shopping and preparation routine went into chaos. Don's food habits and my food needs were completely opposite, like Jack Spratt and his wife, except that we didn't lick the platter clean—we found it difficult to share meals at all. While he could eat my food, he really didn't like most of it. I had enough energy to fix my own food, but not enough to fix two completely separate meals for him and for me. Don also frequently worked late, so he wanted to eat at a different time than I did. The result was that we were each fixing our own separate meals, except for the sharing of some vegetables. Mealtimes as a time for sharing and bonding became much too rare.

No sugar? I attended a Ph.D. celebration for one of the people in our Tai Chi class and happened to sit at the table next to Sifu. The next day, I went to Tai Chi and my joints were all sore and locked up. When I complained to Sifu, he said, "Well, that's not too surprising, considering what you were eating."

"Really!" I said. "So what was I eating that is causing sore joints?"

"All that sugar," he said.

"What? I didn't even know I had any sugar."

"Yeah! Those Thai noodles had a lot of sugar in them. Also the sauces. It goes straight to your joints, locks them up. Try laying off the sugar and you'll get better."

Sugar too? My list of "noes" was getting longer than my list of "yeses!"

Nevertheless, I laid off the sugar—no more afternoon Snickers bars, no more pies and cakes—and, lo and behold, my joints felt better! I was gradually learning what effects all kinds of different foods have on my particular body, even though I still didn't know why I responded in this way.

Food Shopping and Cooking. The food shopping also went through transition. We no longer needed large quantities of food, but Don was still in the food-throwing mode, so we would wind up with large quantities of the wrong type of food in the pantry that no one would eat. In the fall a mouse family came into the apartment through a crack in the living room baseboard and tried to relieve us of this problem. We had more mouths to feed than before, but of the rodent variety. They had a feast on the uneaten food, and we had a big mess. Ethel, our housekeeper, salvaged what she could and carried it out to her church's food pantry. The mice knew they had a good thing going and didn't disappear until we rehabbed our apartment and plugged all the holes.

Because of the different types of food I needed, we had to shop at different stores for at least part of our groceries. It was much easier to be sure about the contents and quality of the food if we shopped at Whole Foods, a health food supermarket, so we began trekking up to the north side of Chicago for our shopping trips. Whole Foods pledges not to shelve items with unnatural substances in them and to label all produce as either "conventionally" grown or "organic." While the food at Whole Foods is wonderful, it took a while to get used to all the new terminology and the new types of food, such as all the varieties of tofu, bean products, soy products and bulk foods. I began buying high-protein grains we never heard of before, such as quinoa, millet and amaranth, as well as quinoa and rice pastas and more exotic items such as miso and seaweed.

The types of food were one big change—the prices were another! Don was shocked by the checkout bills and began to call the store "Whole Paycheck." After all, we had *three*! sons in college. At first, he felt that the food was expensive enough that he could not afford to eat it, so we shopped in different stores for our food, with him getting most of his food from the local cooperative. He could no longer purchase my food for me because he had no idea what to buy, so, as my strength improved, I began doing my own shopping. Even so, he had to go with me, because I was not able to lift the bags into the car or get them into the house once I got them home.

Learning to cook with the new foods required new cookbooks and a lot of experimentation. At first the food tasted really bland and awful. The classic response of "Tofu? Yuch!" was a daily litany. Fortunately, there were some bright spots emerging in support of the new diet. My Tai Chi friends shared recipes, and when we got together for a potluck we would learn about each other's methods of making tasty foods. Sean began dating Emily, who was a good cook, and from them I got tips on herbs and spices and ways to use sprouts and other fresh foods. Chandler, the son who ran the organic market at Oberlin, lived in a campus vegetarian co-op in which everyone had to help prepare the food, so he developed great skills in this arena. He started doing part-time chefing at a local vegetarian café and became a fine cook, delighting in fixing wonderful meals that satisfied even the most diverse needs and tastes. Eventually three of my sons and one daughter-in-law, in addition to me, became vegetarians, so we outnumbered the meat-eaters in the family—who would ever have thunk it!

Eating Out. Restaurants were a real challenge—no more steakhouses and rib joints! Nowadays, many restaurants in Chicago have a few vegetarian items, but it's still not that easy to get vegan food. Once again, the Tai Chi crowd came to the rescue. We shared ideas on where we could go and what we could get, with Bruce usually leading the way to new possibilities. There are a few vegetarian restaurants in the Chicago area, and I enjoyed going to them because I liked having a broader choice available that suited my needs. Even so, it was hard to find places where Don and I could both eat happily. The best possibilities are Thai restaurants, which will often prepare food with substitutions and may be willing to make special dishes to specifications. Chinese restaurants can usually fix a stir-fry with veggies and tofu, but frequently it is rather bland because they depend on fish sauces for flavoring. Pan-Asian restaurants are a good possibility and also the ones where you select your own ingredients and toppings and they stir-fry them for you.

The search for good restaurants outside the urban area of Chicago was like seeking the Holy Grail. The Midwest was a vegan wilderness. Most foods in buffets and salad bars have meat broth, creams and cheeses in them. Even though I could get a baked potato or salad at many places, I soon realized I needed to carry my little portable grocery wherever I went if I wanted any protein. When going away for a few days, I would take a carry-on suitcase with all kinds of dried foods, canned foods, almond butter, special breads, snacks, and supplements. I discovered some shelf-stable convenience health foods that helped me survive in a beefeater's world. On road trips, Don and I became expert at spotting the type of strip mall that is likely to offer a natural food store.

Fitting in with Family. Back home again in Indiana, when the vegetarian Yorks came to town it was, once again, like the aliens landed. My extended family lives in a farming area, and my brother-in-law, as well as all the neighboring farmers, uses traditional farming methods, including various pesticides and chemicals, to raise his crops. One of the projects he enjoys most is raising beef cattle, so grilled steak and burgers are the company fare. Going hunting for game was also a traditional male bonding experience in the late fall and winter. One can see that eating vegetarian *and* organic was philosophically and pragmatically a foreign concept in this environment. Why would anyone do that?

Nevertheless, there was good-hearted consideration from folks down on the farm. The Tofurky I brought to Thanksgiving dinner was greeted with raised eyebrows, but a few hearty souls bravely tried it and pronounced it "not bad." There was even some amusement at the Tofurky jerky wishbone. Even with the best intentions, however, it took a couple of years before folks could think about holding the cheese on the salad or holding the chicken back from the stir-fry to be added later. My father, who was in his nineties, never did get used to the idea that I didn't order bacon or sausage with my eggs when I went to the restaurant with him. He would shake his head and look over his glasses down his long nose, squinting as if to be sure it was really his daughter sitting across from him.

All the dietary changes highlighted the fact that food is at the core of life. All kinds of axioms apply—if we don't eat, we don't live, we are what we eat, etc. Beyond axioms, we were learning that diet is connected not only with health and survival, but also, very powerfully, with our personal sense of self, our emotional well being, our economic status, our sense of identity and belonging to our families and social groups, and our ties to our culture. When you eat differently from other people, you mess with the biggest things in life.

I think that's why Don would periodically revert to the scientific paradigm in the futile hope of getting things back on a "normal" path. Every now and then he would look at me in frustration and say, "There's no scientific evidence any of this will work!" As my health and mobility improved, I would respond, "Well, look at me. I'm one." That's when Don began describing me, somewhat humorously, as "five sigma," a term which means that something is non-statistical, is unlikely to occur in the real world, and comes as close as science will allow to being a "miracle." We were learning that there are some people in the world who just don't fit into statistical patterns and that those who don't fit them have to seek diligently for their own unique paths to healing and wholeness. Unfortunately, that can be a little uncomfortable for people around them!

Walking Free

It was late August in 1997, and I was taking advantage of the cooler morning hours to do Tai Chi in the little park in my hometown, Worthington, Indiana. Some senior citizens were walking briskly around the circular paved track that enclosed the park, and they gave me some curious glances as they made their rounds, wondering what kind of strange movements I was doing. People in this little rural town had never seen a live demo of Tai Chi, so I gave them a nod and a wave to assure them I was friendly. Dogs often wanted to investigate me, especially when I was hanging upside down, and on some occasions children would come up and just stare at me until I stopped and answered their questions. On this day I wanted to be alone.

I was thinking of my mother. She had suffered from Parkinson's disease for several years, and her once vibrant personality and boundless energy had deteriorated until she was physically and mentally a shadow of her former self. Now she was in the hospital, and we all knew her time on the Earth would be short. My older sister needed to take a trip to Alaska to attend to her family, so I drove myself down to Indiana. It was a mark of my improved health that I was considered able to care for my father and to stand daily watch at the hospital, making crucial decisions regarding her care. Her once-robust form had dwindled to ninety some pounds. Her once-strong limbs were now stiff and were pulling her body more and more into a fetal position. Her eyes, once dancing with light and enthusiasm for living, were now dull and questioning. Only during prayer and the singing of hymns did her eyes light up and one could tell from the loving, faraway look in them that she was seeing her beloved Jesus; therefore, we prayed and sang with her often.

Unfortunately, she developed a deadly, highly contagious virus while in the hospital and had to be kept in isolation. Anyone entering her room had to wear a gown, mask and gloves, restrictions that kept us from ministering to her as fully as we desired. Infection was risky for my elderly father and also for me because I knew that MS attacks can often be triggered by viruses. Nevertheless, I took the risk, armoring myself with gowns and masks and lots of prayer and faith. Due to the restrictions, I was the only one who was going in to see her for some of her last days—and then only for short visits. It was a sad vigil, but Daddy and I did our best to keep each other cheered and to comfort Mother as best we could.

When I finished my Tai Chi in the park, I felt refreshed and comforted. I sat on a picnic table, sipped some water and took in the peaceful scene. The field across the fence was full of new-mown hay, and the fresh, pungent smell brought back memories of my childhood on the farm. The shade under the giant oaks and maples was cool, and there was a gentle breeze that stirred the air now and then. Soon the morning dew would be gone and the day would be getting hot. I sat there for a while, thinking of my mother and what an incredible person she was. At the most difficult times of my life she had been there for me, supporting me, encouraging me, inspiring me. I sent up little prayers for her. "I love you, Mother. You're going to your beloved Lord, dear Mother, your struggle is almost over. Peace is coming to you, and freedom, freedom from all the pain. I love you, Mother."

Tears trickled down my cheeks, and as I wiped them away, my attention came back to the little park where I was sitting. I looked at the bandstand a few yards away where my wedding reception had been held thirty some years before. I remembered how it looked festooned with the multi-flora roses my sister had collected from the roadsides early on the morning of the wedding. I looked at the shelter house were my parents had celebrated their fiftieth anniversary, and I remembered the festivity and joy of friends and family. The place was full of memories, good memories, memories that can strengthen, inspire and invigorate. It was a place of new beginnings and celebrations. I reached for the handle of my black, ergonomic metal cane, thinking I would walk over to the bandstand. I stopped for a moment and looked at that cane. I had been wanting to walk without it but just hadn't got up the courage to do so. I looked around at the small park and sized up the situation. The paved circle was not too big, and there were benches along the way where I could sit and rest. My car was parked nearby, next to the shelter house, and I knew the people were friendly and would help me if I needed assistance. Hmmm. I paused for a moment. Yes, I would do it. I took a deep breath, laid the cane back down on the bench, and headed for the track. I was going to take a walk.

A cane was my friend and constant companion for many years, but eventually, as I healed and gained strength, it became a liability. I was accustomed to keeping the cane with me at all times, even when I used the electric scooter, because it helped me in shifting from the scooter to a chair or to the car, and it gave me stability when going short distances on my own. As my health improved, I used it on my walks around our residential park. It was difficult to go straight forward when I was walking because my left side was very weak and all my weight tended to shift to the right. I also carried the cane in my right hand and leaned on it for support. As a result, my torso twisted to the right and threw my body out of balance so that I tended to head for the bushes on the edge of the sidewalk. It took a lot of energy and concentration to constantly re-direct myself.

I discovered that dependency on the cane not only oriented me to the right but also gave me a downward and forward, torqued orientation. I bent downward with a curve in my shoulders and back, causing a shortening of the muscles in the front of my body and in my hip flexors. The tight, shortened muscles made it impossible to stand up straight, so I expended unnecessary energy trying to hold myself erect and prevent myself from falling forward as I took each step. The downward orientation was exacerbated by my habit of focusing my attention on the ground in front of me. I was so afraid of falling that I was constantly watching for obstacles or uneven places that would cause me to trip.

Bruce recognized all these imbalances and began showing me how to correct them through exercise and regular bodywork. He would do bodywork, cranial-sacral therapy, myo-fascial release and whatever else he felt was needed, and then he would give me exercises to build the muscles so I could maintain the new postures. Occasionally he would mimic my gait and posture in a hilariously exaggerated way so I could get the idea what I was doing wrong. I needed to strengthen the left side and stretch the right side so it could come back up to a more normal position. Sometimes the exercises were frustrating and even painful, and I would cry as I was doing them.

While I was engaging in this straightening process, I went to see a behavioral optometrist, Dr. Jeffrey Getzell, a doctor who specializes in the way vision affects performance of various activities such as standing, walking, reading, and writing. Dr. Getzell's tests revealed that I had a very narrow field of focus, somewhat like viewing the world through a long tunnel, with only a small bit of light and color at the other end where I was focusing my eyes. He prescribed lenses that would help open up my field of focus. He explained that balance and coordination depend on binocular vision and that if I would look forward and consciously take in the scenery and activities around me, my balance and coordination would improve. He instructed me to walk as much as possible and to look all around me, not at my feet.

When I took my first walk with the new lenses and followed Dr. Getzell's instructions, I had a shocking experience. First, I discovered that if I lifted my eyes and looked forward, my entire body tended to straighten up. Then my feet could swing through more easily, contributing to a smoother, more natural gait. As I looked up and out, a whole new world opened before me that had been closed off by my narrow focus on the ground in front of me. I could see trees and sky and the faces of people who were passing me. At first this was downright scary. It was almost as though I had been in a protective visual shield that shut me off from the world outside myself. Now such a large amount of information was coming at me that I suddenly felt exposed and vulnerable. This was coupled with my fear that if I didn't look at my feet I would trip and fall. It took faith to believe that following Dr. Getzell's instructions would really help me. It also took a lot of practice. My eyes were not accustomed to the new patterns, and it was almost like learning to see all over again. As I tried to put the visual practice together with walking, my body's balance and coordination changed almost daily, requiring highly focused concentration. I was not able to talk and walk at the same time, so if someone was accompanying me, I had to stop walking in order to have conversation. It was literally true that I couldn't walk and chew gum at the same time.

Throughout all this straightening and visual re-training, I began to realize that the cane was inhibiting my progress. At the same time I was trying to go straight forward, it was pulling me to the right. At the same time I was trying to look upward and outward, it was pulling my vision down toward the earth. At the same time I was trying to become strong and independent, it was a sign of my weakness and dependency. Furthermore, the cane created emotional stress. People who cared about me and were concerned about my safety, especially Don, urged me to use the cane so I would not fall and injure myself—but I wanted to throw it away, even though I was afraid to do it. Now, here in this little town with the smell of new-mown hay, the place where I grew up, the quiet, gentle place I knew from childhood, the place where I had started life with Don, I had courage to try.

Each day, between times when I was attending Mother in the hospital and caring for my father, I would take walks in the town park, sharing the time with Mother as though she were there with me, walking and remembering, encouraging me as she had so often throughout my life. Go ahead, you can do it, Mother always believing in me, walk straight, Mother singing hymns in the morning, keep your eyes up, Mother praying, look at the world around you, Mother's beautiful blue eyes, take longer steps, Mother taking food to a sick family, don't drag your feet, Mother fixing a quick dinner for twelve, keep a steady pace, Mother leading music at the nursing home, you can do it, Mother doing everything with joy, just a little further, Mother's boundless energy, one step at a time, Mother leading the way, each step a praise, thank you, thank you, thank you, keep on singing, singing all the way, singing, walking, leaping, flying, here we go, all the way up through the soft scented air, all the way up through shining green trees, all the way up into the warm morning sun, floating, sailing, rising, rising, all the way home.

We did not have a typical funeral for Mother but more of a celebration of her life, her joy, her service, her spirit, her humor, her love. On the day of my mother's celebration I was walking free with no cane, a phenomenon no one noticed because they were so focused on the events of the day. But Mother and I, we knew. We were both walking into a new life, and we had taken the first steps together.

A Traditional Chinese Medicine Diagnosis

Autumn has always been my favorite time of year, a time when I love to sit outside in the sun under a blue sky, feeling the cool, crisp air and watching brilliant red, yellow and orange leaves flutter down to carpet the ground around me. Somehow, even in the city, I seem able to detect the smell of dried cornstalks and stacked clover hay that I remember wistfully from my childhood on the farm. The knowledge that the glory of the season is the last flame of life before a harsh, cold winter makes it a bitter-sweet experience, one in which I savor each golden, sunlit moment, knowing it could possibly be the last before the damp and cold set in for many long months. During the years of my illness, the bitter-sweetness of autumn also extended to my health. While it brought me relief from the debilitating heat of summer, it also inevitably heralded a dangerous time during which I usually experienced an MS attack. Statistics show that more MS attacks occur during the change of seasons in fall and spring than at any other time, and this was my pattern for many years.

When I returned to Chicago after my mother's celebration in the fall of 1997, I came back walking free of a cane, but I soon began to experience one of the classic MS attacks that accompanied the season. My normal pattern would have been to decline in mobility and function for several weeks, experiencing paralysis and pain, to stay in that condition for several weeks or even months, and then to begin a long recuperation that might be interrupted by yet another attack. This time I was in such pain that I resumed use of the cane and even resorted to the scooter a few times. I went hobbling to Tai Chi class one evening and Sifu Bruce asked, in his matter-of-fact way, "What's going on?"

I replied sheepishly, "I'm having a "neurological event," my way of avoiding the confession that I was having an MS attack.

He said, "Nah! It's the weather."

"Hmm," I said, feeling I had just heard one of the craziest explanations for an MS attack that I could possibly imagine. "Really. The weather. Hmm!"

"It's dampness," the Sifu said.

"Dampness?" My eyebrows emphasized the question mark. "What is dampness?"

"Dampness in the body," he said. "It happens when the weather gets cold and damp. Everyone I work on has it now. I'll give you some herbs, and it will clear it right up."

"Hmm," I said again, wondering how anyone could have the gall to say that what I was going through was caused by the weather. If so, why didn't neurologists know about it! Then I remembered that I was talking to the man who had said, "Nah, it isn't in your head, it's in your hip!" and had unparalyzed my left side using his skills of bodywork. I had better pay attention. He handed me a couple of bottles of herbs and told me to take some immediately and then to take three of them three times a day. "Yes sir!"

To my astonishment, I was completely back to normal in five days!

I checked the bottles of herbs carefully. They were both traditional herbal formulas put into pill form by a company called Health Concerns. One was "Drain Dampness" and the other was "Mobility 2." Astonished, I realized I had been given a diagnosis and treatment according to Traditional Chinese Medicine (TCM) that was a key to my improvement. Right away, I knew I had to find out what "dampness" is.

I began asking around and friends recommended a book that changed my life—again! They suggested I read Paul Pitchford's book, *Healing with Whole Foods*. This remarkable book at first seemed formidable because it uses the language of TCM to describe various health conditions. However, it also connects the TCM to expert descriptions from the Western medical tradition and relates it all to healing methods based on whole foods, herbs and natural remedies. As I read, I began to understand the Eastern tradition from a Western perspective, and this, in turn, helped me grasp my own condition and needs.

Pitchford describes "dampness" as any overly wet or moist condition in the body, whether it is from the environment, poor diet or internal organ weakness. Dampness can manifest as various types of mucoid deposits or growth of yeasts, viruses, putrefactive bacteria, amoebas, and/or parasites. Symptoms are difficult movement, numbness, damp swelling or edema in any part or all of the body, excess mucous that affects the heart and lungs, feelings of heaviness, lack of appetite, bloated abdomen, watery stools, and a coating on the tongue that is thick and possibly dirty or greasy. Pitchford describes certain chronic diseases as having characteristic dampness, including cancer, *multiple sclerosis*, AIDS, chronic fatigue syndrome, rheumatoid arthritis, and other virus- or microorganism-related degenerative diseases. This TCM diagnosis of dampness and the mode of treatment with diet, herbs, and certain mineral supplements became the linchpin of a program that would make huge changes in my health over the next few years.

Pitchford says conditions of dampness are often deeply situated in the body and are not easily resolved by either traditional or modern medicine. Nevertheless, he says there are certain common threads running through these conditions. One is that many of them have yeast excesses in the digestive tract and respond to a diet that is not dampness inducing; that is, a diet that is low in fats and mucous-forming food and high in whole, unprocessed vegetal foods. Exercise is also important because it oxygenates the body. He offers an illustration of a damp cloth that does not mold if it is hung out in circulating air.

I began treating myself for dampness, using Pitchford's guidelines. Since one cause of dampness is *C*andida yeast, I investigated literature on how to eat to reduce *Candida*. My daughter-in-law, who has Crohn's disease, was already way ahead of me. She recommended Jean Marie Martin's book, *The Candida Diet*, and I began following her recommendations. By this time I had read enough about diet to know that this diet was so healthy and clean that it was likely to address many different types of problems besides *Candida*. Healthy eating certainly wouldn't do me any harm!

In addition to implementing a dampness reducing diet, I read Stephen Cooter's book, *Beating Chronic Illness*, which describes how molybdenum, a common, inexpensive trace mineral, metabolizes the acetaldehydes that are produced in the body by the *Candida* yeast. These acetaldehydes can pervade the body, especially after heavy usage of antibiotics, creating all kinds of havoc, including symptoms of many diseases that are hard to diagnose and treat. Cooter's book has a scientific paper in the Appendix that explains the chemical action of molybdenum in dispersing the toxin and suggests an appropriate dosage. Molybdenum is already present in common foods but not in enough quantity to initiate a detox. A bottle of molybdenum was only about $5 at the health food store, so I decided to give it a try. What did I have to lose? I added that regimen to the rest of my healthy diet.

As soon as I took the first molybdenum tablet my body began to detox, ridding itself of many years' buildup of toxins from antibiotics, drugs and poor diet. I sweated copiously, detoxing through my skin and also through urination and feces. I became the incredible shrinking Anna. Puffiness and swelling in various parts of my body began to reduce as excess moisture was released with the toxins. I began losing weight, much of it through excess moisture built up in the tissues of my body. My feet, which had grown from size 9 ½ to 11 ½ over several years of MS, returned to their original size because of released fluid from my tissues. I slimmed down, wearing smaller sizes of clothing and shoes. Over a period of two years I lost 35 pounds and went from wearing sizes 14-16 to sizes 6-8. At the same time, my energy level improved greatly, and the pain in my muscles and joints diminished. My skin cleared up and took on a healthy glow, and many of the wrinkles disappeared. Sifu, who uses skin tone and color as an indicator of health, began commenting on my youthful appearance. I stayed on a strict diet for well over a year and continued the molybdenum until the symptoms of detox were gone.

Jaw dropping became a common phenomenon for people who had not seen me for a while. Most people had only known me when I was in a wheel chair or scooter. Now they saw me standing up, walking around with no cane—and, on top of that, I was looking slim and trim and several years younger! Even sophisticated folk often forgot themselves. They would look at me, and, as recognition dawned, their jaws would drop and they would unabashedly stare me up and down from head to foot, a somewhat disconcerting experience for the object of the voyeurs!

Funny anecdotes began accumulating. I went to a celebratory dinner for a Professor in the Astronomy Department and sat next to a woman a little older than I. My specially prepared vegan meal arrived late, as usual, causing some people at my table discomfort about starting to eat their meals. I encouraged them to go ahead because I was accustomed to such delays because of my diet. When my meal arrived, I began to eat and suddenly noticed that the lady next to me had stopped consuming hers. She had her elbow on the table and was resting her head on her hand, staring straight at me with wide, question-mark eyes. When I glanced her way, she said, "How do you do it?"

"Pardon me?"

"The adolescent skin. How do I get mine to look like that?"

I laughed, amused by her candor, and said, "Well, I imagine it's got something to do with my diet."

She looked at my plate of vegetables and rice. "So why are you eating *that* way?" It was a direct question to ask of someone you barely know, but it was a question that would become common in the next several years when I was eating with people who did not know me well. I then began to explain that I had been seriously disabled with multiple sclerosis and that my diet change had been at the heart of a big change in my health and appearance, including my skin. The forkfuls of food going from plate to mouth began to slow down as the people close to me engaged with the story and registered their amazement.

Finally, the lady next to me said, "Well, that's amazing. That's wonderful, and you really do have beautiful skin. I wish mine could look like that." Then, with somewhat a tone of regret, she continued, "But I don't think that's my route to a gorgeous body. I like my food a little too much for that." At which point, she put her fork into her pasta and, with little enthusiasm, continued eating her high-fat Italian meal. The "adolescent skin" became a little joke among my Tai Chi friends, most of whom were much younger than I. They would say, "Wow! How can I get that adolescent complexion!"

My success in detoxing and my improved health and appearance testified not only to the importance of the diet that had come through TCM but also to the benefits of Tai Chi. In his description of ways to treat dampness, Pitchford describes oxygenation as important and describes several ways to oxygenate the body. The most fundamental are those that one can do naturally through exercise and diet. In the exercise arena, he mentions physical activity, regular exercise, yogic breathing exercises and visualizations to circulate energy. I was already doing most of these through my practice of Tai Chi. Now I understood yet another reason why Tai Chi was so good for me. The disciplined breathing was not only building my energy but also fighting viruses and helping eliminate the anaerobic environment that allowed Candida and other bad bacteria to thrive in my body. I was literally airing them out of my system.

TCM not only improved my physical health but also had an important effect on my ways of thinking about who I am in relation to other cultures. I, being a Westerner from the most powerful nation in the world, had always assumed that our culture was the greatest and most powerful, not only because it is free and democratic, but also because it has the best to offer in terms of science, medicine and technology. Living in the liberal and intellectual environment of Hyde Park, I had participated in many discussions of the downsides of Western cultural imperialism. It was only when Western medicine failed me and I received healing through the wisdom of an ancient, foreign culture that I began to realize in a personal way (rather than a theoretical or philosophical way) the profound gifts of life that can flow from cultures other than my own.

While I had been interested in China for many years and had prayed for the nation for many years, it was from a position of assumed superiority. I had negative attitudes toward China because of its politics of oppression, which I deplored. The Eastern culture was strange and impenetrable to my Western mind. Their ancient religions were complicated and mysterious. I had regarded China as being in need of Christian evangelism. I had failed to see the depth of the Chinese people's struggle to survive and come into full function in the modern world, and I had failed to understand the negative impact Western culture has had over many years on the economics and politics of eastern nations. Now my personal life was touched and I was being healed through their gifts. The prayers I had prayed with sincerity but ignorance were returning to me on waves of healing. I was the one who was being evangelized. My mind and heart were opening with appreciation and thanksgiving for the Chinese people and for the blessings that were coming to me through them.

Drug Free!

"Don't go off the Betaseron. If you do, statistics say you will revert to your previous pattern of relapsing-remitting exacerbations. It's better to deal with the side effects." It was my doctor, Barry Arnason, speaking to me on the phone. I called him to tell him how much difficulty I was having with the drug. It was making me ill every time I took it and was causing joint and muscle stiffness and arthritic pain. I listened carefully to his warning and hung up the phone feeling frustrated. I was making progress in my healing, but I wasn't ready to depart from what I viewed as the security of the drug, even with its painful side effects.

It is extremely difficult, intellectually, emotionally, culturally, and financially, to venture out of the dominant paradigm of Western medicine to seek healing in alternative and complementary therapies, at least it was for me. All my life, and especially throughout most of my illness, I relied on traditional Western medicine to diagnose my physical problems and treat them with the latest high-tech equipment and drugs. The assumption and expectation that this was the proper thing to do—the only thing to do—was so deeply ingrained that nobody I knew questioned it. It was almost like the "One Way to Heaven" doctrine I learned when I was growing up. One dare not stray from the true path at the jeopardy of one's life.

Most Christians I knew expected healing to come through the medical channel. For as long as I can remember, most prayers for healing were connected to God's will, which was expected to work through medicine, with God "guiding the hands of the doctors." Thus, doctors and medicine were integrally tied into our theology, prayers and spiritual practice. It was almost like doctors were a specialized type of priest who took care of our bodies while the priests in the churches took care of our souls.

The God of Western medicine is Science. In church we committed our spirits to the God of Abraham, Isaac, and Jacob; in our doctor's offices and hospitals we paid homage to Science. Science is the miracle worker in our culture. The power of Science has been so great that many people have decided to follow the Science god and scrap the one found in church, who doesn't seem very powerful in comparison. Science has all the answers, which can be discovered through careful research, controlled experimentation, peer-reviewed analyses and grants from the NIH. If Science doesn't reveal the answer now, we expect it soon will. For this reason, we pay careful attention to the latest research results, as though they are revelations from on high—even though the results tend to change every few weeks.

I have had my share of blessing from Western medicine, and so has everyone I know. I wouldn't be alive without it, nor would many of my loved ones, and I am grateful for all it has done for me. Andrew Weil, the guru of healthful lifestyle at the University of Arizona has said, "If I'm in a car accident, please don't take me to an herbalist." I feel that way too. The science and technology of putting people back together after severe injury is astonishing. Science has also brought into usage some of the powerful drugs that are giving people relief from many afflictions, including MS.

However, even with all its "miracle" cures in so many arenas, it has not been able to heal many diseases, including my own. I followed the current wisdom of Western medicine and Science, according to the most expert of its practitioners, not knowing about alternatives and being discouraged from following them if the questions came up.

"No scientific evidence" dismissed for many years any inclination I had to experiment outside of conventional practice. Many alternative and complementary therapies are not accepted because there is not yet enough rigorously researched data available on their efficacy for various populations of people. Those who want to try such therapies take the risk of spending their time, energy, money and health on products and procedures that may be ineffective or even harmful. Since I resided in the same house with a scientist and in a community that highly values science, there was a strong, built-in resistance to doing anything "unscientific." Don viewed my whole healing enterprise with the skepticism of one who wants to see hard facts and who wants to have a body of double-blind, peer reviewed research behind every procedure. He felt that if herbs are so great, the doctors would know about it. He has a lot of faith in scientific medicine and he didn't want me to do something that would be harmful to me.

He had a point, of course. The threat of charlatans gives added sting to any inclination to explore alternative therapies. Sophisticated but unscrupulous quacks are ready to take advantage of desperate people who will try almost anything to alleviate their suffering. Some horror stories from the patient perspective are documented on the website of the National Multiple Sclerosis Society. I didn't want to be a victim of such schemes. An acquaintance of mine recently revealed the dangers to me from a different angle.

I met Dr. Komer (not his real name) in the health club in our building. We were often working out on the treadmills or doing floor exercises at the same time, and eventually we struck up a conversation. He noticed my hard work and dedication and also that I was making progress with my rehab. When I told him my story, he listened respectfully and was impressed, even though I learned that mine was not initially an easy story for him to accept. He is a Harvard-trained pathologist who did some consulting for a company in the Chicago suburbs that claimed to have a remarkably effective therapy for healing multiple sclerosis. While he is normally skeptical of such claims, he did some digging and discovered that it was funded by federal grants and other reputable organizations and that it had passed federal inspections. As far as he could tell initially, it seemed to have solid scientific data to support its claims.

Dr. Komer is a compassionate man and wanted to investigate the possibility that there might actually be something available to help people with MS. The company hired him as a consultant to investigate the authenticity of its claims. To their chagrin, his expertise revealed without question that they had manipulated their data in extremely sophisticated ways to show positive results when in fact they were a total sham. People had been paying thousands of dollars for a worthless therapy. As a result of his investigation, federal authorities shut down the whole operation. Unfortunately, as the company crumbled, its founder made an attempt to salvage it by falsely claiming that Dr. Komer was a Director of the company. The Federal government blacklisted him for three years from holding the directorship of any laboratory, and his sterling career was locked up in red tape and placed in jeopardy. Other reputable doctors were hurt as well, eventually shutting down the work of physicians with over 100 years of cumulative training and experience. I was astounded to hear firsthand how far some people would go to make money by cheating vulnerable, innocent people—and how hard it is to detect them and shut them down!

Besides issues of scientific credibility, financial concerns were also a big deal for us. We had great insurance coverage through the University that included doctor visits, hospitalization and drugs, but it didn't cover less conventional practices, not even chiropractic treatment. Our budget was tight, and we couldn't just decide one day that we would direct a couple of hundred dollars a month toward supplements, herbs, and bodywork. We had to gradually fit it into the budget until we were able to make long-term changes to accommodate the extra expense. Financial commitment didn't come easily, especially when there was no "proof" that it would help.

I moved into every new thing slowly and carefully, observing how my body responded to each change. Sifu Bruce never encouraged me to stop taking medication, knowing that my body was very sensitive and that changes needed to be undertaken with caution. He listened and observed and concentrated on building me up, not on getting me off drugs. He also insisted that I keep careful records of how my body responded to every new therapy.

As I moved more and more into use of herbs, nutrition, bodywork and Tai Chi, I was faced with the question of whether to stop using medications. As I felt better and better, I gradually discontinued use of some of them. With each one I watched carefully for some weeks to see what the effects would be. If I continued to improve, I felt it was safe to leave it behind.

The thousand-pound gorilla was Betaseron. My doctor was one of the lead researchers for this drug, which was the first one that was documented to change the course of MS. It was proven statistically to reduce the number and severity of exacerbations for patients who fit a certain profile. I went on this drug in 1995 and responded in a statistical fashion with fewer and less severe episodes. Even though it had positive effects, reactions began to build up over time until they became quite severe. For a long time, I thought my symptoms, including stiff, aching muscles and arthritis, were part of my disease. I used my herbs and other therapies in a complementary fashion, alongside the Betaseron, for over three years.

In the spring of 1998, there was a glitch in my prescription that caused me to go off the medication for about a month. During that hiatus, I discovered that it was the medication that was making me ill. When I stopped taking it, I felt much better. I talked to my doctor three different times, and each time he insisted that I should tolerate the side effects and repeated the warning that most of those who go off of the medication return to their previous frequency and severity of exacerbations. It was very scary for me because I wasn't sure my immune system was strong enough to do without the drug. It was even scarier for Don, who was so skeptical about all my "unscientific" therapies anyway. I had gained some ground, and he didn't want me to lose it.

In the summer of 1998, a severe toothache hastened the decision. We were in Oregon attending my niece's wedding when excruciating pain developed in my jaw. I couldn't tolerate that pain and also the pain caused by the medication, so I stopped taking the Betaseron. I didn't contact my doctor because I knew what he would say. I just decided to take really good care of myself, follow my dietary and exercise regimen and believe I would be okay. I was fearful about what would happen in the autumn, which was the season when I would traditionally have a severe MS attack.

When autumn arrived, so did the symptoms of an MS attack. I handled them successfully with herbal therapy and my health continued to improve. Even so, because MS is such a capricious disease, it took me months to feel assured that I was in fact doing okay without the drugs. As I progressed successfully through the dangerous winter and spring seasons, my hope and confidence grew. I began to trust my body and to trust the decisions I was making. I was able to say tentatively to myself, "I *think* I am drug free."

Drug free! For me, departing from the faith and practice of Western medicine was like putting my soul in jeopardy, not to mention my body. Today alternative approaches are more in the popular awareness, with about 30% of the population having tried them in some form at least once. The economic crisis in our country has caused many people to seek alternative approaches, and the internet and media have made yoga and Tai Chi more familiar and accessible. Throughout most of my life and illness, however, they were unheard of, kind of like those suspicious Eastern religions. As a matter of fact, the connection of many therapies with Eastern culture has often made them seem not only foreign and medically questionable but also spiritually suspect as well, at least to people in my conservative circles. It took careful thought and preparation and a lot of hard work to go off of drugs. Afterward, there was continual re-evaluation and often fear and doubt. I was stepping outside the circle of paternal safety, committing myself to the big, threatening world of unscientific possibilities. I was stepping out from under the protective arm of the HMO into independence. I was taking responsibility for myself and believing in myself, a very scary enterprise indeed!

Over time, my confidence has grown. Now it has been many years since that momentous day in 1998, and I can say confidently, "Yes! I am drug free!" I am well and strong and growing stronger day by day. I now take responsibility for myself and have confidence in my decisions. I explore the options available to me and make my own decisions. I am grateful for medical science, but I no longer feel it is God. Science is good and valuable for the service it renders, but it is not omnipotent.

My disease and my healing all began in a different day and a different time when I was a different person. I had a smaller, narrower view of the world and of God, and that smaller view constrained my ability to reach out into the unknown and unfamiliar to find healing. The healing process opened up my perspective on the world and that in turn caused me to see a bigger God. I learned that God can use all kinds of people and all kind of methods to bring us healing. It is not the practice itself that is "godly" or "not godly." It is our faith and trust in God that leads us to seek out those methods that God knows will be the most effective for us, even if they are not the most common or familiar. After all, Christ himself was an alternative healer, working outside the accepted Jewish system of healing laid down in the Mosaic law. That's why they kept throwing him out of their synagogues and ultimately crucified him.

In spite of our fears, in spite of the financial pressure, in spite of the quacks and charlatans, those of us who are "incurable" need to open our eyes and our hearts, to search without ceasing anywhere and everywhere, inside and outside ourselves, for the answers we need, for the answers that are certainly there as God's gifts to us. Perhaps, indeed, we are all "incurable" and need to engage this search. Perhaps in medicine, in life, in God, we will discover an exceeding, infinite abundance of merciful, loving, healing, hopeful, bountiful possibilities.

Body Prayer

The struggle to find a balance between doing and being has surfaced again and again since my experience of sudden head-to-toe paralysis when I was thirty-seven years old. Before that time, the question of balance between the doing and being aspects of life never even occurred to me. I was a flat-out, plain and simple hard-core doer. I defined my worth by all the things I could *do* for myself, for others, and for God. I spent my first 36 years doing, doing, doing, buying into the achievement syndrome that is at core of the American Boomer character. When paralysis struck, my "doing" core was deeply frustrated. I spent several years bashing my head up against the outward achievement wall and falling back, weak in body and wounded in spirit. Then, during the years of increasing disability, I began to turn inward, finding power for living in meditation and prayer. Eventually those meditations and prayers became outwardly manifest, first in prayer ministry and then in the larger ministry that led to ordination in my church community. Finally, in the time of deepest paralysis and weakness, I came to a place where I felt completely fulfilled in *being*, entering into a mystical relationship with Christ and expecting that I would die and be raised to walk eternally with him. During all this time, my spiritual life was disconnected from my physical body and health except to pray for healing and expect God to answer those prayers in some mysterious, mystical or miraculous way. I didn't connect the condition of my spiritual health with my physical health. I thought I was a perfectly healthy spirit that for some unfathomable reason was imprisoned inside a disastrously dysfunctional body.

Now, as I was in the process of co-creating a new life, taking responsibility for myself, actively pursuing healing through exercise, diet, and disciplined lifestyle, I also understood that my previous spiritual life had always been out of balance, either toward doing or being. I had been like a swinging pendulum, never able to settle into a truly healthy integration of these seemingly antonymous dimensions of life. In my conservative, fundamentalist religious context the spirit was for worshiping God and the body was for doing the will of God. It was a dualistic separation that in some way reflected our dualistic ideas of good and evil, transcendent and immanent (God out there and God in here), creator and creation, them and us. I had never integrated the physical and spiritual parts of myself, had never got them both up and running and healthy at the same time. Now I discovered that I needed all my resources pulling in the same direction. I could not heal without "getting it all together," body, soul, mind and spirit. Instead of focusing on doing and/or being, I needed to focus on *becoming* whole.

My practice of Tai Chi began to help me get it together in ways I could not have anticipated. This happened as I began to practice building chi, not only in the Tai Chi class and in Tai Chi exercises and form, but also in my daily practice of healing, including physical exercises, meditation and prayer. As I practiced taking chi into my body through my breath, I also began to think of it as taking the life of God into my whole person, body, mind and spirit. When I thought of chi flowing in my body, I thought of the life of God flowing in me, healing me in every part. I began to seek out and practice ways of integrating meditation with physical practice.

Breathing. All of the meditation methods I used incorporated breathing in some way. No matter where I was or what I was doing, my breath was always with me. By conditioning myself to focus on my breath, I could more quickly become centered and peaceful. Because the breath carries life-giving, healing oxygen to every cell of the body, it is an excellent way of visualizing life and healing flowing into every part. In addition to the focusing and calming effects, it also energized me, resulting in a feeling of refreshment and strength. Thus, I discovered that this "Eastern technique" is powerful for people of any faith and from anywhere in the world because it employs and enhances a basic function of life. I experienced that disciplined methods of breathing are God's gift of love to all people through the Eastern cultures.

Visualization. Most methods of meditation I used also incorporated some sort of visualization, which could take a variety of expressions. While I had used visualization for several years, such as in the "Picture on the Way," that visualizing had been more intuitive and was accomplished mentally and spiritually, not as an integrated practice with my body. Thus, it was a kind of "transcendent" visualization, usually picturing God outside myself or as only in the spiritual part of myself, which I felt at that time was the most important part. Now I intentionally practiced a more "immanent" visualization, picturing God in every atom, cell, muscle and bone of my body, through breath, blood, nerve impulses, muscles and energy.

Many years previously, when I experienced the "Baptism of the Spirit," I had felt a wonderful, warm river of the Spirit pouring around and through me and had felt greatly energized. Due to my dualistic framework, I had thought of it as a "Spiritual" event, not one that could empower me physically and holistically. Thus, the experience had been one of those unsolved mysteries of the spirit. I didn't know what it meant or how to use it, so many of the benefits were lost. Incorporating the idea of "chi" helped me understand that the spiritual experience could energize me physically as well as spiritually. I began to think that I could have that kind of experience again with more understanding and hopefully with more skill and wisdom as I put it into practice. I began to feel that the Spirit was more and more integral to every aspect of my being.

The Spirit of God is expressed in a variety of images in the Bible, including wind, water, and fire. "Chi" is often manifest as warmth or heat in the body, so I visualized the flame of the Spirit in my innermost being, physically associated with my abdomen, and then, using the technique of the micro-cosmic orbit that I learned in Tai Chi, I would breathe and circulate the chi around my body, causing the heat of the flame to permeate my whole being. Sometimes, incorporating the idea of chi, I visualized the Holy Spirit as water, starting at the top of my head and flowing down in me and through me, a wonderful, river of the Spirit. As it flowed, warmth would flow through my whole body, energizing me and bringing life to my cold limbs. In this way, the breathing and circulation of chi was not only a physical and spiritual discipline but also a means of healing for my whole person. In keeping with the core Christian idea that Christ became incarnate in a human body, I called this kind of practice "incarnational meditation" because it integrated my whole self, body, mind and spirit, into experiencing the life of God. Eventually, I began to call it "body prayer."

Body Prayer. For too many years I was immobile. Now my body needed to move and come to life, and I learned to move during meditation as well as in physical exercises. In fact, exercise became meditation and meditation became exercise. I found many ways to integrate movement and meditation.

Chi Kung is a series of slow, deliberate movements designed to increase and balance the flow of energy in the body. Chi Kung is a powerful mode of meditation in itself, but some styles lend themselves especially well to meditation because they incorporate visualization of such archetypal elements as wind, breath, water, birds, sun and moon, rainbows and other natural phenomena. One of our Sifus, Ed Gierut, frequently leads a "Set of Eighteen" that includes many beautiful, inspiring images, accompanied with expressive flowing movements that represent the image and that also open the "meridians," allowing a fuller flow of energy. The result is a feeling of lovely, calm refreshment and nourishment of body, mind and spirit.

Some of the Chi Kung movements, such as moving the hands in and out with each breath, worked well as breathing exercises for self-healing. For example, I would draw the hands in during an inhale, drawing in life, breath and healing; then I would move my hands away during an exhale, breathing and pushing out anything that is harmful or impure, including negative emotions. I also used these motions when praying for the healing of other people.

Visualizations of Christ empowered much of my meditational movement. I would get calm and centered, breathe regularly and focus my attention on my center of gravity in my abdomen. Then I would think of myself as moving from that center, which I identified as Christ in my innermost being. The challenge was to originate my movement in the Christ at my center and keep my attention fixed on Christ, no matter what, whether I was walking forward, backward or doing any of my many exercises. This focus calmed my emotions and gave me a sense of divine presence, empowering me to do exercises that otherwise seemed impossible. Body prayer was becoming a powerful mode of healing that integrated every aspect of my life.

We often think of prayer as something that is done with the mind while the body remains passive or assumes certain static positions such as bowed heads, folded hands or kneeling postures. Body prayer is based on the idea that when we come into God's presence we bring our whole persons and that our physical bodies are an integral part of the selves that we present to God.

Body prayer recognizes that we address God not only with feelings and thoughts but also with motion and body imagery. It proclaims that we communicate with God not only with outer expressions and movements but also in our innermost beings, our organs, tissues and bones; not only with vocalization but with the processes of breathing, blood circulation, elimination and other body functions. It declares that we speak to God through our bodies and that God speaks to us through our bodies. The communication among body, mind, and spirit in God's presence becomes a magnificent Dance of Life which calls us into harmony with ourselves, with each other, with all of nature, and with God.

Eventually, I put the meditation and the traditional healing movements of Tai Chi and Chi Kung into a Genesis creation story setting that I could do as a combination of meditation, worship, healing and physical rejuvenation. I did it alone to begin with, but after some years I did it with other people too, and we discovered how deeply satisfying it was to do the healing movements in the context of our own spiritual heritage. The creation movements became a bridge between cultures and faiths that began to purge my doubts about my experience even more than theology and doctrine. When it became worship, I knew I was becoming deeply harmonized with my healing.

Mental practice. As my rehabilitation progressed, I was often exercising two or three times a day for perhaps twenty or thirty minutes, and in between I would be thinking about what I had done in the session or what I would be doing the next time. I discovered that I could enhance my workouts by doing mental practice. Mental practice involves thinking into my muscles and imagining how they would move, how they would feel when performing certain activities, how they would work together to achieve the results I envisioned. Mental practice works in both forward and reverse modes. For example, after I finished a workout, I would recall how my feet felt when walking the balance boards, how my legs felt when they were in line with my feet, and how my body felt when shifting weight and trying to stay balanced. Then, when I was imagining as clearly as possible, I would think about how I could change a movement or posture so it would be more effective. I tried to imagine as closely as I could what it would feel like if I were doing it correctly, thinking of myself as straight and strong and steady. Along with imagining the physical, muscular sensations, I would also imagine the emotions and perceptions I might have while attempting certain exercises, emotions such as fear or frustration, and I would try to think of replacing them with positive feelings. Often this imagining would give me an insight that I would put into practice during my next exercise session. In this way I could make progress even when I was not actually engaged in exercise! Much later I discovered there is a solid body of research showing that mental practice is effective because it stimulates all the same areas of the brain as physical practice. The fact that the mind is able to do some of the work while the body is resting is great news for people who struggle with low energy.

Affirmations. Affirmations were important to my daily practice of meditation. Long-term disability instills a deeply ingrained sense of all the things that are impossible. Over a period of years, certain normal activities dropped like rocks into the fathomless depths below the surface of daily life, never to appear again as real potentials in my life. Walking, running, sitting up straight, opening heavy doors, crossing the street, playing musical instruments—so many important and beloved activities were lost. After a while, the hurt of the loss became numbed and I lived without the activity or skill as though it never existed. There were so many things saying no to me as a person with disabilities that it required a strong positive intentionality to move past the status quo and regain an old skill or create a new one. I exercised this intentionality through the use of affirmations—statements of "I can" and "I am able" and "I will" in a myriad different forms:

> *"I can walk this hall straight down the center."*
> *"I can cook this meal myself."*
> *"I can step up on this curb."*
> *"I am able to lift this leg just a little higher and do it one more time."*
> *"I have the courage to make this trip alone."*
> *"I will do this even if it seems impossible."*

Performing even the simplest actions in everyday life required that I become a constant source of inspiring conversation for myself. I could be my own worst companion by constantly whispering little "no-nos" in my own ear, or I could be my own best cheerleader and boost myself to the next goal, giving the lie to everything and everybody who said no. I chose the cheerleading role. I had new challenges every single day, and affirmations gave me strength and courage to tackle each one.

I AM Identifications. "I AM" identifications are statements of unity with the attributes of God's character, life and action. For many years I had been interested in the myriad names of God and had compiled a very long list of God's names, which I would study and use for meditation. I knew that all the names together still do not express the fullness of God but only point in God's direction. Nevertheless, I knew that it was very important to know the names in order to call upon the one that is appropriate for a particular situation, enlivening my faith for that aspect of God to be manifest in my life. I learned over the years that in their most powerful form I AM identifications could become a decree that God's life will be manifest in a certain way, such as in Faith, Hope, Love, Light, Joy, and Healing. I AM identifications of this kind had been at the core of my "Rising Manifesto" that gave me courage to live through the darkest time of my life. At that time I had used them mostly for spiritual healing. Now I began to use them for practical healing of my whole person.

I discovered through a friend that the Jewish Kabalistic tradition is alive and well today and that there are Kabalistic meditations that incorporate most of the elements I needed. The Kabalistic approach fit me well because of my love for the Hebrew language and my long study of the Hebrew Scriptures, including the many names of God. The Kabalistic approach includes a chart of the names of God and a repetition of "I AM" names, with each name associated with a particular part of the body. The names include Wisdom, Understanding, Strength, Beauty, and Compassion, among others. I would say an "I AM" name, accompanied by breathing and by placing both hands on the associated body part. As I did so, I identified myself with that attribute of God, bringing myself to awareness that it is God's life working in every part of me.

I used different names at different times. "I AM light" helped me experience God's light as part of my being; where there is light there can be no darkness, no illness, no weakness. "I AM life" identified me with God's life which I could feel flowing in me anew. For many months I almost exclusively used the one that would bring me from death back to life, the same one that Christ declared just before he raised Lazarus from the dead. He declared, "I AM the Resurrection and the Life!" Time after time, I repeated this identification, in every activity, every exercise, with practically every breath I took, waking or sleeping: "I AM the Resurrection and the Life." This affirmed to me that in all my parts, body, mind, and spirit, I was rising from the dead to walk in newness of life. Death was falling away from me like the grave clothes from Lazarus' body, like the shroud from Christ. I was being set free by the power of God's life in me. I was decreeing life into myself and my world by declaring myself to be one with the Rising One.

As I gained strength for myself in meditation, I also gained strength to pray for others. Private prayer and prayer with other people became less a litany of hopes and requests and more a declaration of faith. I was able to visualize God's activity in healing, saving, rescuing, and guiding other people through the trials of their lives. I visualized the physical breathing that accompanied my prayers as breathing the life of the Spirit into each person's life and situation. Instead of calling for God to be present, I practiced thanksgiving for the ever present I AM, active at all times, never failing, always full of love, wisdom, and power.

The being-doing dilemma has been at the core of my healing for many years, and I know now that the dilemma is resolved not by choosing one or the other or even by finding a balance between them. Rather, it is resolved by giving myself completely to the process of *becoming* all I can be, all I AM. In order to engage that challenge, I must understand that I am and I AM incarnate, just as Christ was incarnate—that the body is the temple, the house, the home, the fully infused habitation of the Spirit. Nothing I do in this world for God or with God will be done without my body. When my body is gone, my work in this life will be finished. I must cherish this body, heal it, love it, care for it, so that my body itself is a prayer expressing the fullness of who I AM.

Detoxing the Emotions

The process of healing from my long disease exposed depths of emotion that I had never suspected were in me—fear, anger, shame, sorrow, horror, panic, mourning, frustration, hurt, disappointment—the built-up emotions of many long, painful years. Just as my body had held in the toxins for so many years and was now cleansing itself through healthy diet, exercise, and herbal therapy, foul emotions that had also been held inside began to come out for cleansing and healing.

The emotional purging worked in tandem with my physical healing. I didn't know at that time the chemical mechanisms or how the brain processes the messages, but I experienced the practical reality that emotions are stored in the tissues, muscles and bones of my body. This was surprising to me because I, as a product of our Western culture, was accustomed to separating emotional and bodily illnesses into different compartments. After all, medical doctors work on our bodies, and psychiatrists and psychologists work with our emotions and psyches. Doesn't that mean that they function separately? This compartmentalization is in contrast to the Eastern healing arts, which treat the person as a holistic unity, assuming that body, mind and spirit are all intertwined. When the body is hurt or healed it affects the mind, spirit and emotions as well.

I discovered the body-mind-spirit connection experientially when I began healing through the Eastern arts. As I began working certain muscles again that had not worked for years, memories of pain and emotions connected with that part of my body would come out, and I would experience feelings almost as acutely as when an event had first occurred. I did not know until years later that motor neurons are connected to memory centers in the brain, thus explaining how exercise affects the emotions. The most common feelings I had were connected to the process of deterioration as MS consumed my body and my life. As I activated a muscle for the first time in years, I would have the memory of when that part of my body first failed me, of my pain, my grief, my loss, of the mourning for a part of my life that was dying.

Thus, the healing process was a time of strong emotions. Several times I experienced side effects in certain parts of my body from medications I had taken years earlier, and my thoughts would go directly to that time and the feelings connected with taking that particular medication. It seems that residues of the drugs had been locked into my tissues and organs and were being released, along with poison emotions, through my sweat and tears. Bruce repeatedly assured me that this was part of the healing process. "It's all coming out. Let it go, girl. Better out than in." It did seem that these emotions were coming up for a last review before their permanent departure. I became accustomed to acknowledging the feelings and the hurts, declaring them to be in the past, and saying good-bye to them forever.

Emotions would often be purged out during Tai Chi class. All the body's parts are moved during the exercises, and as muscles are activated that have been inert for many years, emotions tend to be triggered and come up for examination. Sometimes I would work through the Tai Chi moves with tears streaming down my face. People in Tai Chi class were accustomed to such things happening and responded with understanding and compassion—sometimes they were the ones doing the crying.

Emotions also came out during bodywork sessions, which I had with Bruce every four to six weeks. Each of the meridians is associated with a particular set of organs in the body, and each set of organs is associated with certain emotions. For example, the gall bladder meridian is associated with anger, the spleen meridian with pre-occupation of the mind, and the kidney meridian with fear. Sifu Bruce could sense and feel the energy in the meridians and could tell when they were "blocked." For years my gall bladder meridian was blocked and the muscles running along it, especially in my right hip and leg, were stiff and painfully fiery to the touch. He would manipulate that meridian and the muscles in that area, saying, "You're blocked up there.

You have some anger in there." I also had a lot of pain in the spleen meridian, and he would note, "That's preoccupation. You've got a lot on your mind. Just let it go."

The fact that I had these emotions was often news to me until the energy was unblocked. Then the emotions would begin to pour out, and I would be confronted with my true feelings. Those feelings were not easy to deal with. It was like talking out my problems in deep psychoanalysis, except that it was my body doing the talking in a language too deep for words. It is unfortunate that I did not learn this language much earlier in life, because my body was wiser than my intellect. As the emotions were acknowledged, expressed, and purged, there was a feeling of release, often accompanied by deep relaxation of muscles. In turn, relaxation and a sense of well being from increased endorphin production relieved pain and allowed me to progress with exercises to improve my mobility. Thus, the healing of emotions was integrally related to my physical healing.

As emotions began to come out of hiding and I experienced how they contributed to crippling my body, I recognized that I needed to make changes in the way I handled my emotions in order that I could heal more effectively—and not make myself sick again! I realized I needed to learn to express my emotions in healthy ways. Unfortunately, I didn't know how to translate my insights into action. Patterns of feeling and behavior ingrained throughout a lifetime are not easy to change. I had to intentionally decide to be more honest and forthright in expressing my feelings, and I had to decide how I would deal with the reactions from other people who were unaccustomed to this new mode of expression.

Don was the one on whom I "practiced" my new emotional honesty the most. I was surprised at the anger that began to emerge toward him, especially because I knew in a rational sense that he had done the very best he could throughout my long disease. I "scape-goated" on him because he was the most convenient person on whom I could vent. At the same time, there were issues that had been in our marriage for many years that had affected me deeply while I was ill, feelings that I had long repressed and denied or that he had rationalized away when I expressed them. Those emotions needed to be cleared.

There were also emotional issues surrounding Don's work. He was the Founding Director of the Sloan Digital Sky Survey, an ingenious project designed to map the Universe. At the same time I was doing intense healing work, his project was in financial straits, and there was one crisis after another. Solving crises had been a daily part of Don's life for many years, but this one was the *Mother of All Crises*. The pressure was overwhelming. It threatened to wreck all his hard work, his professional integrity, his self-image, and—from my point of view—our relationship as well. I felt that Don's professional crises were like waves that continually rolled in on the shores of our lives. No matter what happened, the waves would keep rolling in. Now they seemed to be thundering breakers. I couldn't delay my healing process until they were finished thundering, because I felt that would never happen. I expressed my feelings—another way of saying I turned my emotional guns on Don.

My new mode of communication felt like "et tu Brutè" to Don at a time when he was beset by many foes. I was the beloved and trusted friend who joined in the fray, my words piercing to his heart like daggers and making his plight seem more desperate. He began to sink under the pressure of all the stress at home and in his job, and his health deteriorated. I was angry that he was not taking steps to take better care of himself. No matter what he did, I found fault with it. My emotions put him into a lose-lose dilemma.

I was getting emotional help and support from friends, but Don had a manly aversion to seeking such assistance, so the pain dragged on. After his big crisis was over, he needed a long healing period at the same time I was healing. Our closest friends saw and sensed our interpersonal tensions. They had seen Don support the family with suffering for many years, and now it looked to them as though I was ungrateful and unsupportive of him. They couldn't see the deep but painful healing that needed to occur in Don and me, not just as individuals, but also in our relationship. For that reason, they tended to move more toward support of Don, at the same time opening some distance in their relationship with me. I am sure their perception of my unjust attitude played a role in the gradual deterioration of my status as "Saint Anna." A practical principle in such cases is to refrain from entering into too-swift judgement. It took years before Don and I each healed enough and re-developed enough confidence in our love for each other to communicate more honestly and effectively.

Roaring and Forgiving

I was in our living room praying with a young woman in our small group, an exceptionally talented, vibrant young woman who eventually went to seminary and is now co-pastoring a church in California with her husband. She was sitting at my feet with her head in my lap, and I was bending over her with my arms gently around her shoulders. When we finished praying, she lifted her head and looked around with a puzzled expression on her face as though she were listening for something.

"Did you hear that noise?" she asked.

"What noise?" I said.

"That loud noise, like a gale, so strong it was shaking the windows."

"No," I said, "it's perfectly quiet in here. When did you hear it?"

"I heard it when my head was next to your torso." Then she looked at me with big, round eyes and said, "It's the roaring of the centuries."

The emotional pain from years of disability and from hurt relationships seemed huge, but there were other layers of emotion that proved to be just as important. Those deeper, more hidden levels revealed some of the root psychological factors that no doubt contributed to the origins of my disease in the first place. Perhaps it was in those deeper levels that my friend heard the "roaring of the centuries."

I struggled all my life with the stigma of being female. From the time I was a child, I felt the pain of being restricted in the ways I could serve God because of my gender. Traditional patriarchal interpretations were manacles hanging from my hands and feet, and I was so accustomed to them that I thought they were a normal mode of dress. I wore them into the 1960s, a time when feminist issues were seething. I didn't burn bras, march in the streets, divorce my husband or become a lesbian theologian. Even so, I was not isolated from the spirit of the age, and I began to explore my own questions about my nature as a female person.

While we lived in Princeton in the 1970's, I spent three years researching and writing my own feminist theological manifesto, using the outstanding library resources of the Princeton Theological Seminary. I was an amateur, but I plunged into the subject with my customary gusto. I worked my way through textual and critical arguments surrounding Old and New Testament passages. I read history of the church's position on women, including the offensive statements by early church fathers who blamed the fall of the human race on females. I read nearly all the feminist theology available at the time—there was not nearly as much of it then as there is now!

I came to personal convictions that were strongly counter to my evangelical upbringing, concluding that God created male and female to be equal partners, both in the first creation and in the new creation brought into the world by Christ. I came to believe that the church has lost its original vision of all people being equal in God's eyes. Even while I tended my house and my babies, I was privately moving beyond the fringes of my traditional church interpretations, a ship sailing quietly out of the harbor to the open sea. I began to feel good about myself as a woman, and I was proud of being created female in God's image. Even so, my circumstances at the time did not allow expression of my inner convictions. Through many years, I repressed my strong feelings and sought modes of ministry and service to others that were within the framework of evangelical acceptability.

Eventually a price must be paid for years of bearing injustice and repression—of any kind. I paid a price. I discovered that my disease was not just about what had happened in my own personal life but also about the fact that I am a woman. I discovered that my manner of dealing with my emotions and relationships and the activities and aspirations of my life was not just a product of my own personal upbringing but of my nature as a female person. During my healing, I looked back and saw that I had responded to my circumstances in ways that women have always responded, by submission, subjugation and denial of my true self. I had pushed the feelings down into the deep waters of my psyche, and now they were rising up like creatures from a primordial lagoon, gasping for air and fighting for life, declaring, "I'm alive, I'm alive, you can't drown me or kill me or say I don't exist!"

I felt a strong sense of injustice about the way women had been treated in my own lifetime and throughout the centuries. I felt deep personal hurt and outrage, and my feelings moved beyond the personal into the communal and archetypal. I felt I had been chained to the wheel of history with countless other women, women who suffered through the ages far more than I, women who salted the trail of life with their tears, women who tried to break free but who, in spite of their bravest efforts, fell under the crushing wheel and were broken. I felt connected with all those women as though it were I myself who experienced the suffering and injustice through them, as though I were joined in heart and spirit to all of them, no matter what place, no matter what time, no matter what race or age, throughout all history.

Archetypal images flashed on my consciousness, images of women in other times and other places around the world, women who experienced some trauma of womanhood. Some were African, some Asian, some Hebrew, some Arab, some European. Sometimes these women had faces and sometimes they had names. Sometimes I had heard their names before, and I researched their stories and lives, probing deeply into their personalities, motivations, and character. One such woman was Theresa of Avila, the great mystic, who had a long illness in her life that had many of the characteristics of multiple sclerosis. She, like me, was healed of her disease when she was about fifty years old. Another was Judith, a wealthy and beautiful woman whose story is recorded in the Apocrypha. She lost her husband at an early age and lived as a hermit, spending her time in prayer in a little hut on the top of her house. When the enemy of the Jews threatened their land, she dressed up, went into the enemy camp, seduced the general of the army and cut off his head, carrying it back home with her in a basket and saving her people and her land. I identified with her and with others as though they were myself, and, in so doing, I learned many things about myself. I entered deeply into each woman's life, saying, "This is who I am. I am this woman."

Sometimes the women had no identifiable historical personality but seemed to be emotional and spiritual types of women throughout all time that were brought to life by my spiritual imagination. One of the women, an African, had her firstborn child taken from her by her husband to offer as a sacrifice to the gods; I felt her rage and saw the hatred in her face. A Chinese peasant woman's child, a female, was taken by her husband and left in a ditch to die because they could not afford to support a female; I felt her hurt and helplessness in view of her grinding poverty. An Arab woman was part of a prosperous merchant's harem; I understood her politics and her bisexual relationships. A highly educated Chinese woman made a scientific discovery, but it was claimed by her male mentor; I experienced her sense of betrayal and helplessness in being manipulated by a man. Another Chinese woman, much-loved by her father, died at an early age of a genetic disease that had already taken the life of her mother. A Jewish girl was highly talented in her studies of Torah, but her less capable brothers were the ones who became rabbis.

As each of these women came into focus in my consciousness from the realms of imagination and collective unconscious, I experienced her hurt, hopelessness, passion, despair. It seemed I was each of these women. It seemed, in a sense, that I was Woman. I would often feel anger toward the men who caused their pain, and sometimes I would feel a profound but helpless rage at the underlying male-dominated "system" that locked women into their fates. The "system" included politics, social mores, cultural practices and yes, of course—religion. I had a great deal of still-unresolved anger that religion had oppressed women for so long when I knew in my heart that women were created as equals with males. I became more and more sensitive to God-language in the Bible and in prayers, hymns, liturgies and other religious settings and learned to "think double" in such situations, being highly aware of the way things were being said and silently translating into God-language that was more inclusive, even when I was not free to express that language. I became more aware that the very language we use locks us into oppression. The "system," for millennia in the past, formed the background for the suffering and oppression of women that occurs around the world today. In a sense it is the "system" that made me sick, my disease being a horrifying metaphor of our crippled, broken human condition.

Anger toward the "system" is deep and cannot be resolved by one individual, certainly not by me, nor can it be resolved in one lifetime. The "system," by its nature, is always there, is always flawed and is often evil; it is always in need of redemption. As I discovered, however, healing can occur that gives hope, courage and faith to engage the struggle as it exists in our lives now and in the lives of those around us.

I looked at my own life and reviewed the way the hurt of the centuries had been redeemed in some way by the men in my life. I remembered my gentle grandfather, who had been a great spiritual guide; my loving father, who had inspired me with his ability to continually grow and transform; my sons, who had opened me to new and strange things and thus brought so much healing to my life; my mentor and friend Shanta; my healer and helper, Sifu Bruce; and so many others. Most of all, I thought of Don, the man who had been my heart's friend and companion, the man who had been with me through everything, healing and hurt, for better or worse, richer or poorer, my partner, my love, the core of my life for nearly forty years. Yes, we had our problems, but the magnificent fact remained—he was still there, through it all!

I thought of him and the others, and my potent anger began to be assuaged. I reflected that each of these men is human and each struggles with his own flaws. At some time I have felt hurt by each of them, either personally or by the way they function within the "system." Nevertheless, each is good in heart and spirit. Each of them fights the "system" in his own way, seeking justice. As I acknowledged my emotions and purged them, I also was able to acknowledge that the "system" does not just oppress women but also men. It keeps all of us from fulfilling ourselves as we can and should, as we long to do. When the humanity of some is denigrated, so is the humanity of all. I was not just Woman, I was also Man.

As I thought of the remarkable men in my life, my heart began to soften. I knew that I have seen in my own lifetime the answer to millennia of hurt and suffering—the answer of Love. I saw the hurt redeemed in my own life in a thousand different ways, and when I saw it, I began to forgive. Over time the forgiving began to bring a release, almost as though I were forgiving not only those in my own life but also the world, forgiveness like a healing stream, running through the millennia, flowing in, around, and through me.

Perhaps all of this emotion was the "roaring of the centuries" my friend heard when she was praying with me. Thus did it roar through my life like a raging lion and pass on through as a lamb of forgiveness. Forgiveness brought healing of body, mind and spirit. Even so, I knew that the fact that I had forgiven did not mean that the oppression in the world would go away or that my hurt through other women would be finished. It meant that I would commit myself to a new dimension in that struggle, one of healing instead of hurt, forgiveness instead of anger, hope instead of hate.

"Chi" and Other Dilemmas

Healing was a multidimensional experience that was happening concurrently at every level of my being, but I could perceive and focus on only a tiny portion of the healing process at any given moment. For a long time I was consumed with the physical aspects of gaining strength, balance, and control over my body. Emotions intervened at various times, and of course social dimensions demanded my attention. As my healing progressed and my life took a different shape, I was aware that some essential intellectual and theological questions were rumbling in the depths and that one day they would rumble to the surface. My mode of healing was too radically different from all of my previous experience for me to let it go unexamined. I began asking the question, "What does it mean?" even though I knew the answers would not be easy and would take a long time, perhaps the rest of my life, to become clear. The questions were scientific, philosophical, and theological. At first many of them centered on the "chi" in Tai Chi. Chi was powerful and real for me because I was experiencing the flow of chi in my own body and it was healing me. But I needed to get the experiential into dialogue with the intellectual and spiritual aspects of my being. I needed to make sense of what "chi" is and how it relates to my own Western scientific context and to my own Christian spiritual tradition. I wanted to know, "Is there anything in the Bible about chi?"—because, after all, the Bible had been my reference point for my whole life. It would help me understand where I have been and where I am going.

The talk about meridians and acupressure points and energy centers sounded strange and foreign to me. I had no idea at first whether the terms were just metaphors or whether such things as "meridians" really exist. When I mentioned "energy" and "meridians" to Don, he was quite put off. As a physicist, his definition of energy had very specific, measurable qualities. As for meridians, he dismissed them as being unscientific and unprovable, foreign to the Western medical paradigm and therefore without credibility. If I continued to pursue these ideas, it would not be with the blessing of mainstream science.

I read widely on my own, not only within my own Biblical tradition, but also exploring the writings and spiritual practice of people from other traditions, both Christian and non-Christian. I probed works by theologians such as C.S. Song and Diana Eck. I read a wide variety of writers on spirituality all the way from Brother Andrew to the Jewish Kabbalists to the Buddhist Thich Nat Hahn to Thomas Merton, modern Christian healers, Yogi Ramacharaka, Paramahansa Yogananda, Rudolph Steiner, and Lao Tzu. I also read books by contemporary energy healers and practitioners of therapeutic touch. Bruce gave lectures each year as part of Tai Chi class that helped to explain various aspects of the theory and practice. Gradually I began to put together a picture, even though at first it looked like a jigsaw puzzle with a lot of missing pieces. Shanta, with his wealth of personal experience and theological expertise, helped me explore how the Bible could speak to my questions and how I could relate my experience to what I knew of the Judeo-Christian tradition.

According to Chinese philosophy, chi is the life that permeates all things in creation. Humans are born with some chi, which they get from their parents, and they have their own chi, which they take in through the air, water and food they eat. Without chi, nothing can exist and nothing can live. We need to maintain the "chi" energy we have and also build our energy so that we are able to function well and be healthy. Sifu explained that chi flows through the body in "meridians" or "channels" to all parts of the body, including not only the external parts through which we sense and move but also the internal organs, such as liver, kidneys and spleen. Chi can be blocked by tension in the body so that the energy cannot flow freely. Sifu explained how the meridians are opened by various Chi Kung and Tai Chi moves and how the energy flowing through these channels supports better movement and health. Every now and then he would make a reference to the "energy centers" of the body. He said that "Tai Chi" means "grand ultimate" because it has to do with using, building and controlling the energy that sustains all things. To practice the "way" of "Tai Chi" or "Tai Chi Tao," is then to practice the "grand ultimate way," improving and progressing toward one's potential as an integral part of the whole creation.

Eventually I concluded that chi, as I was learning about it, is part of everyone and everything; it is part of the way things are. Just as we all have hands and feet and lungs and livers, everything that has life also has chi; therefore, like hands and feet, lungs and livers and any other part of the human person, chi is morally neutral. It is not having a hand or foot that makes one moral or immoral, good or bad, a Christian or Hindu; it is what one does with one's hands and feet and other parts. Just as one expresses individuality through choices and usage of the body, one can also do so through choices and usage of chi. The neutrality of chi seemed to be a reason why people from every religious background and spirituality, including Taoists, Buddhists, Jews, Christians, and Muslims, could feel comfortable in our Tai Chi class. We were each personally exploring the meaning of what we were learning and using it in our own unique ways. The principle of neutrality of chi came through also in martial arts films such as *Crouching Tiger, Hidden Dragon, Hero,* and *Fearless,* in which both the good guys and the bad guys all use their chi, each according to his character and intent for good or evil.

Shanta, helped me explore how the Bible could speak to my questions and how I could relate my experience to what I knew of the Judeo-Christian tradition. Once I started looking, there were many connections. In Genesis when humans are created, God is described as breathing into their nostrils the breath or spirit of life. It seemed to me that this life was possibly another way of talking about chi, a life force that originates with God and inhabits all living creatures, both animals and humans. Throughout the Hebrew scriptures, breath, air and wind are all characteristic of living creatures. While breath is ubiquitous, it can carry either positive or negative energy with it, depending on the character of the person. For example, before Jesus ascends, he breathes on his disciples and tells them to receive the Holy Spirit. The breath of this holy person conveyed blessing and power. In contrast, before the Apostle Paul's conversion he is described as "breathing out" threats and murder against Jesus' disciples. His breath conveyed fear and danger. These examples, and many others, spoke to me that chi, or the force of life, is present in everyone and that the quality that goes out from each person's chi depends on the character and intention of the person.

I found other similarities as well. When practicing Tai Chi one often feels chi as "heat" or "fire." The upper portion of the central body is called the "upper burner," the middle section the "middle burner," and the lower section the "lower burner." Those who are more experienced can move the chi around to different places in the body at will. Even I, with my limited experience, could warm my body up by breathing from the lower burner. Similarly, in the Bible fire is a metaphor for power, and it can be either good or bad, depending on the person who uses it and the context in which it is used. For example, God's protecting presence was with God's people in a pillar of fire as they came out of Egypt. On the day of Pentecost, flames as of fire sat over the disciples as they received the outpouring of the Holy Spirit. In contrast, fire is a destructive force in times of war and violence. Fire is good or bad, depending on how it is used.

In my Tai Chi group we talked a lot about eating nutritious food as a way of building our chi. Good food can impart good health and life, while junk food produces weakness and leads to disease and death. I saw a similar idea of food as a way of taking in life in both Jewish and Christian writings. The manna in the wilderness appears as a life-giving gift each morning, but it is used by each person according to personal need and intention. The Christian Eucharist consists of food, wine and bread that has been blessed and that contains within it Christ's promise of "This is my body" and "This is my blood." The power of Christ's life is there for all who take it, but each person receives it according to his or her own faith and intention. One may use it as power for living and serving and another may forget it happened.

These comparisons of chi, life, breath, fire and food led me to feel that chi is not a religious concept but that it is a term describing something that is common to all human experience. It is so fundamental and so pervasive that people around the world have developed their own unique ways of talking about it. It is called "spirit" and "chi" and "qi" and "ki" and "prana," "ruach," "pneuma" and many other names. It is humanly universal and morally neutral. It is the morality and character of the person who is using it that gives it a direction toward good or evil.

I continued my exploration. I knew from my experience in Tai Chi that when we were sensing and feeling energy, we were experiencing the human energy field or what many people call the "aura." The energy field is not very familiar and may in fact seem weird and "occult" to people in our culture, especially those who come from a conservative background similar to my own. But the energy field is taken as a matter of fact in many other cultures.

I looked for evidence of the energy field in the Bible and found it with no difficulty at all, even though it wasn't called that. One of the best examples is the story of the woman with the issue of blood who touched the hem of Jesus' garment and was healed. At that time Jesus felt energy go out of him, even though she did not actually touch his physical person. She was touching his energy field, and his energy field had so much power in it that she was healed without his prior knowledge or consent. Jesus, who could sense and control his own energy and use it for any purpose he desired, felt the change in his energy and knew someone had touched him.

There are many instances of Christ and the apostles laying hands on people and healing them. Some healings occurred by giving a person an item such as a handkerchief that had been in contact with an apostle, and some occurred when a person came into the shadow of an apostle, indicating an area of energy around the healing person. We western Christians have so thoroughly westernized our ideas of Christ that we have forgotten he lived in an Eastern context in which such things may have been taken much more for granted.

I thought about the many great paintings of Christian art that depict halos or a glowing aura around the body of Christ, the apostles and saints. I had always thought it was just an artistic way of representing their holiness. Now I began to think that the halos could be a stylized way of showing the energy field around such individuals.

I also recalled stories in the Hebrew scriptures of people such as Elijah and Elisha, who healed by means of objects that belonged to them or by touching or lying on a sick or dead person. It began to occur to me that the ancient practice of laying-on-of-hands was not just a ritual of faith but also a mode of conveying healing energy. These people were holy in character and practiced their healing with great compassion. No doubt their holiness was a source of their healing energy, and they knew how to focus their "good energy" and direct it to dispel the "bad energy" of disease and even death. It occurred to me that what we were learning in Tai Chi class was the nuts-and-bolts aspects of the ancient healing mode of laying-on-of-hands. It seemed that when we were doing healing work, we were using the energy of the human energy field, along with faith, compassion and love, to achieve the healing. I recalled Pentecostal meetings I had attended in which those gifted in healing would bring their palms toward a person, not necessarily touching them, and that sometimes the person would feel such power that they would fall down. I understood that they were intuitively focusing their energy while they exercised prayer and faith, asking the Spirit of God to move through them.

The idea that the use of chi might be operative in Christian healing came home to me in a practical way one morning when my African-American housekeeper came to work. She said, "Oh, Miz York, I'm feelin' so bad today." Dorothy was one of my greatest spiritual supports. She came three times a week to help with everything from laundry to cooking and cleaning. But her most important ministry was her prayers. She was a mighty prayer warrior, a holy woman of God, praying and singing her way through my house, cleaning it physically and spiritually, bringing in blessings, comfort and love.

Dorothy was a soul partner. She would sometimes come into my sunroom-office, lay her hands on me and pray in a rhythmic, melodious croon: "Jesus, we thank you Lawd, thank you Jesus. You're here right now, right now, Lawd, yessuh, you're a good God, you're a mighty God, we're thankin' you God because you hear our prayers, yes Lawd, you hear us. And you goin' to answer us Lawd, because you love us. You're with Miz York right now. She gonna be all right, Lawd, yessuh. You not goin' to let her down cause you love her. Whooh! Mighty God! Hallelujah! Bless her! Bless her, I say, right now, right now, bless her Lawd! Thank you Jesus, thank you, thank you, thank you." Then she would take me in her big arms and hold me close. I would bury my face in her soft bosom as though I was cradled in the arms of God and she would stroke my hair and say, "It's all right now, it's goin' to be all right."

On the morning when she came in feeling low, it was my turn to comfort her. I had no inhibitions with Dorothy. Without even thinking about it, I asked her to sit in a chair in the dining room, and I began to do therapeutic touch in the same way Jeremy and I did with each other, standing behind her to start with and moving my hands in gentle flowing motions out and away, a short distance off the body, praying all the while. I moved my hands from the area of the head, down around the torso; then I went to the front and began again at the head, moving my hands gently and rhythmically, out and away, out and away, praying and loving her all the time. I could feel tense energy become calm, as though the flowing gestures were smoothing a troubled soul. As I moved and prayed, Dorothy began to relax. The tension went out of her face and body, and she began to say, "Thank you, Lawd, thank you, you're a good God, yes Lawd." When I got to her feet, I put my hands on them and prayed that all tension and hurt would go right out through the soles of her feet. "Thank you Lawd, thank you." Then I did a repeat pass all the way from head to toe, gentle flowing movements just off the body, to seal in God's healing.

When I finished, I was behind her, and I put my arms around her as she sat there quietly for a few moments. Then she turned to me and said, "Where you learn how to do that, Miz York?"

I said, "That's therapeutic touch. It's some of what I've been learning. I took a class in it recently, and Jeremy and Sean do it with me. Why do you ask? Is it okay? Do you mind that I did that?"

"Lawd, no!" she said. "I do that all the time, any time I'm prayin' for people for healin', I been doin' that for years."

"Really!" I said. "Where did you learn to do that?"

"I just always did it. Nobody taught me. I just knew. That's what I do. The Holy Spirit moves my hands and I prays for the healin' and God does it. God is good."

"Does anyone else you know do that?"

"Oh, sometimes at an altar call. But we don't talk about it. It's just something we do naturally."

This holy woman, a prayer warrior, healer and helper to many, a good solid Baptist, had no doctrinal hang-ups to inhibit her. She was tapping into an ancient mode of healing that rose up archetypally from her innermost being and that was rooted in her African-American heritage. Out of a heart of compassion she did naturally and easily those things that worked to heal and uplift others. Regardless of the cultural origins of her mode of healing, she had the hands and heart of Christ.

I did not share my struggles and insights at that time with my church. I needed to ground them in a much deeper, broader, textual and contextual study of scripture. The implications seemed profound to me, but I did not have the expertise or the energy to express them at that time. It took all my strength to work on my healing. I held these things in my heart and shared them only with Shanta. We continued our dialogue over a period of at least six years, sharing books, ideas, analysis and interpretations in between our pastoral duties and activities. It took much longer, however, before I could begin to articulate the meaning of the healing I was receiving. For some people who were close to me and were confused about what was happening, it took much too long.

Clearing Out, Moving On

When each of our boys left for college, we asked him to clear out his room to the walls. All garbage had to go, and any personal items or mementos had to be stored in boxes and put in the basement. We needed to rehab the house to keep up its value, and we didn't want to clean out their junk and make their decisions for them. As they went to work, their rooms would belch out prodigious quantities of useless trash that had accumulated in the corners, under beds and in the backs of closets. The condo dumpster could not digest all the refuse, so it would vomit it out into the breezeway in a jumble of cardboard and plastic trash bags, requiring the garbage men to do overtime to get it all in the truck. Sometimes it took hiring a hauler to carry away large items. This was especially true for our oldest son, who was the prize pack-rat of all time. During his high school years, he had collected seven old console television sets from the streets of Chicago. He and his friend had planned to throw them off the top of the building and video them as they smashed on the pavement below. When his parents nixed this enterprise, the TV sets went into the basement for several years, along with a junk refrigerator and other appliances he had stowed in the bowels of the building for spare parts on his building projects. Yeah, it took a truck!

The cleaning-out process for these life transitions was arduous and messy; it was also emotional. Photographs and mementos from childhood would surface, along with the memories attached to them, and there would be stories and tears. "Oh, look, do you remember this?!" "Do you remember when…?" And there were also the inevitable questions: "Can I bear to part with this?" "Will I ever need this again?" Each boy had a hard time deciding what to take, what to pack and what to throw away. I was sympathetic and encouraging but also resolute. The job had to be done because I couldn't deal with all their garbage and didn't want it lying around for another ten or fifteen years.

Unfortunately, I was much better at helping my kids make such transitions than I was at making them myself. Throughout the many years of my disease, I had repeated dreams about houses, which seemed to be an archetype of my body and the structure of my life. Bombed out houses represented my bombed out, dysfunctional body. Exquisitely beautiful houses represented the healthy, beautiful life I wanted but did not seem able to obtain for myself. Houses stuffed full of junk represented things I was attached to but needed to let go. I had nightmares in which I would wander through a chaotic warehouse, probing into mountains of stuff, picking up a few pieces here and there and tripping over refuse in the search for some valuable trinket. Once I dreamed my house was on fire and I kept desperately grabbing things to carry out, barely escaping with my life before all the contents went up in flames. As my healing progressed, my dreams changed. Sometimes I would see myself in beautiful rooms with custom-made furniture, a sign of hope that I was creating a new life. The house dreams always cued me about the status of my subconscious mind.

The house metaphor was manifested externally in our constant struggles with our own condo, a huge old place that required unceasing attention and repairs. We did three big rehab projects over a period of six years. In the process of my healing I cleaned out a lot of stuff, outer and inner. More and more I realized that it wasn't just a few corners or closets or rooms that needed cleaning. I needed to restructure the whole house. I needed lifestyle changes.

Throughout my healing, I was trying to do too much. I was ordained as a minister and was experiencing all the challenges of a new position, new responsibilities, and new types of ministry, along with maintaining some of the old ones, such as leading a small group at my home. At the same time, I was working full time in my market research job. I was trying to fit healing in around all the structural things in my life that had been there before. It was kind of like the time when we first came to Chicago and moved into the big house that was already full of our landlord's stuff, along with all the mice and the squirrels in the attic. It wasn't a good fit. I made progress with my healing, but it was two steps forward, a step back, a step forward, a step back.

It was in early 1998, two years after my initial healing at Tai Chi class, that I completely overdid myself. The stress was so bad that I developed severe shooting pains in my chest that doubled me over. I couldn't stand, sit or lie down without excruciating pain. Don was out of town, so I took myself to the emergency room for examination. I called Bruce from there to get the names of all my herbs in case they wanted to know what I was taking. He was disturbed that I was there by myself, so he called Sean and Emily and then sat and talked to me until they arrived with our mutual friend Chris to keep me company. I will never forget the evening because there in that emergency room a lot of things changed. For one thing, Sean and Emily announced their engagement to be married, and the four of us sat together, eating manna bread and cherishing the sacredness of the moment as we shared the first hours of their lifelong commitment to one another.

As their lives were changing, so was mine. The doctors checked me out, told me it was stress, and sent me home with Tylenol. The next day I had a bodywork appointment with Bruce, and he relieved my distress in a single session with some very painful but effective manipulations. I was grateful, but I knew I needed to make sure this kind of thing didn't happen again. At the next Tai Chi class, Sifu Bruce sat me down knee to knee, looked me in the eye, and said, "You have to make a choice. You can't heal yourself if you go on like this. You have to stop all these things you're doing and focus on healing."

I said, "What do I have to do?"

He laid out a regimen of diet and exercise and said I would have to cut back on my other activities to make space for the new regimen. He said if I would do it, he would oversee my program. I agreed to take on the challenge.

I couldn't change everything at once, but I began working out three times a day, walking on balance boards and doing exercises with weights, bands and other equipment. If I worked out only once, my muscles would forget what I had done and go back to their old patterns. Thus, I was exercising morning, noon and evening, albeit not for very long periods of time, especially at first. I also went to Tai Chi class three times a week, religiously arranging any other appointments around those times.

I gradually cut back my marketing work from 45–50 hours a week to a more normal workload. However, as I was discovering in many arenas of life, healing is a sword that cuts two ways. As I gained in strength, my employer, Diane, began to want me to go with her on market research projects, both in the city and out of state. I didn't know what I was capable of doing, and I wanted to attempt new activities. I also felt I needed to grow with the needs of my job, so I tried new things, usually coming back from my excursions exhausted and needing recovery time. Evaluation of what I was able to do and setting priorities accordingly was a constant struggle and one in which I did not always make good choices.

As I became stronger, my relationship with many people, including Diane, also changed. She is a very strong, dominant personality, a perfectionist, highly motivated, and an expert at what she does. I think there are several reasons why we were able to work together successfully for so long, nearly fourteen years. I was also a perfectionist, and she respected my work. She was proud of the reports and presentations we put out, and she always saw that my needs as a disabled person were met so that I could do my job. From my side, I enjoyed the work, and it kept me up to date with things that were happening in the outside world. I also respected the fact that she was always working on herself, recognizing her own imperfections and trying to overcome them. Over the years, we shared many personal and professional trials and triumphs that drew us together.

Nevertheless, no relationship is perfect, and ours was no exception. When I was weak and disabled, I always submitted quickly to her wishes regarding the work we were doing. After all, she was the boss and the expert. We had conflicts, but I didn't have strength emotionally or physically to push my opinions. A few times when work was slow, I went out and found other freelance work, even though my employment options as a handicapped person were quite limited. This caused her to eventually hire me full time in order not to lose my expertise. These tensions set up a co-dependency under the surface of our relationship that sometimes stirred the depths and occasionally rose up and troubled the waters. As I got stronger, our relationship changed. I began to take a more active role and express my feelings about our interactions, resisting certain behaviors and decisions I didn't like. Sometimes we broke into open conflict, but, more often, we retreated to our corners, nursing our frustrations and strategizing about the next move. Thus, as I healed, another of my most longstanding relationships was changing in ways in ways that were stressful and frustrating.

My employment issues came to a focus in the summer of 2000 at the same time we were thinking of selling our home and moving to new quarters. There was a slowdown in contracts for our marketing company, and it was a financial burden to keep me on staff. Tensions increased, and I decided I would seek other employment. I settled on developing a private tutoring service for students at the University of Chicago Laboratory School and received a lot of encouragement from my friend Chris, who had been doing it for many years. It was a huge step to launch out on my own, but tutoring fit all my criteria for a job. I could do it at home, I could run my own business, and I would enjoy using my teaching and mentoring skills to work with young people. I resigned from my job, to be effective on the first of August. It was a difficult time for both Diane and me as we finished up our last projects. We had shared so much together and were deeply invested in each other's lives. I was thankful for all the experience and good times we had shared, but I felt it was time for both of us to move forward in our own unique ways. We were together for fourteen years. We parted as friends and still share that friendship today.

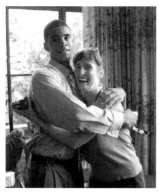

2006: Matt is one of my star tutoring students.

At the same time my job was changing, we also decided to move to smaller, more easily manageable and less expensive quarters. The boys were all gone, we had just finished the third major rehab on our apartment, and it was now in a condition to sell. After much heart searching about leaving the family home, we put the house on the market on the same day I resigned from my job.

Now it was our turn to clean everything out to the walls, throw out the trash, and make the hard choices our boys had to make when they moved out—but we had many more years of stuff to sort through! We decided that the process of selling was stressful enough by itself and that we didn't want to add to it by trying to purchase a home on such short notice; therefore, we decided that after the sale we would find a place to rent while looking for a new home. We hoped to sell by the first of August so we could move and be ready for my new job and for a trip to China in September—pretty tight scheduling.

We did sell our house by September, for cash, and we asked a University real estate person to find us an interim home. She directed us to a high-rise apartment building on the lakefront, a setting that initially seemed strange and unlikely. I was firmly attached to the ground and had never considered living in a tall building. I requested a two-bedroom apartment and did not see the place until a week before we moved in, assuming that I could handle anything for the short time we intended to be there. I was amazed to discover a beautiful, four-bedroom, four-bath apartment overlooking the south end of the lake. It had the added benefit of indoor parking, valet service, a small grocery store, and—best of all—a health club just a short ride down the elevator. I could go down there to work out a couple of times a day with little interruption to my work schedule. To top it all off, we were offered a large rent reduction because they promised a two-bedroom and couldn't deliver on time. I realized this was a place where I could enjoy living for a long time, if necessary. My healing and my changing priorities were causing big, structural changes in our lives, and God was providing abundantly at every step along the way!

Cutting the Strings

The big changes in my life began to create reverberations in my church life and ministry. When I was ordained, I had no role models for how to do ministry as a disabled female, and afterward I had no role models for how to be a disabled pastor in the process of healing. Other people's expectations—and my own expectations—created a special set of stresses, pressing in on every side. I had learned that gaining strength was a sword that cut two ways in my job, and now I discovered the same was true for ministry. The more strength I gained, the more expectations people had that I could do "normal," more "traditional," pastoral ministry. The paradigm of the invincible pastor is very strong. Ministers are not expected to have struggles of their own, and if they do have them, they are expected to subordinate them to the needs of others. Those who set pastors on ivory pedestals inevitably discover they have feet of clay.

I had never done hospital visitation, and I did not consider it a possibility because of my disabilities. Nevertheless, I discovered that some people, including close friends, were disappointed in me when I did not visit them in the hospital when they had surgery or gave birth to a new baby. These disappointments gradually built up over time as I failed to meet the traditional expectations of the pastoring role.

It was difficult being a pastor in a church in which I had been a member for so long. As I gained strength and took more overall leadership, I saw things more and more from a pastoral perspective, prayerfully seeking what was good for the church as a whole, not just for the individuals and small groups within it. I never launched out in making decisions on my own but always submitted my ideas and concerns to the leadership of Shanta, my senior pastor, and to the other members of the pastoral team. I was a consummate team player, never undermining decisions we made as a group. As time went on, personal agendas of those in the church, especially those in the core group, came more to the forefront. Since I was a layperson who became a pastor, some of my friends expected me to make certain changes in the way ministry was done in the church, especially in regard to their own areas of expertise. They felt sure I would make the way for them to take control of their own ministry areas. I was working my own miracles; why couldn't I work some for them? They were disappointed and increasingly frustrated when the changes they hoped for did not occur.

All of this was exacerbated by the fact that I myself was constantly exploring what new things I could do in ministry as my abilities changed. From the outside, my pattern of behavior probably seemed inconsistent and confusing. After all, when I was ordained I was very disabled, and people liked the ministry "Saint Anna" did then. No one knew at that time that I would be healed and had no idea what I would be like in ministry as a healed person. They had no role models for being the congregation of a seriously disabled pastor in the process of healing.

As a matter of fact, pastor or not, no one really knew what the process of healing looked like for someone who had been as disabled as I had been. I looked strong and confident on the outside. They didn't know my hidden struggles. Even my closest friends had no idea of the hours of hard work that were necessary in order for me to make small improvements. It was kind of like none of us bargained for a "process" of healing. We had all read the story of Jesus healing the paralytic, and we had all hoped for an instantaneous miracle like his. But I was an anomaly to the ideal Biblical healing story--mine was a miracle that I had to be working every single day! Even though I had not discussed my theological questions with anyone but Shanta, I did continue my Tai Chi practice, and for some people that seemed to be the "icing on the cake." Since some people felt Tai Chi was a spiritually questionable activity, they raised the question of whether or not it was really Christ who was healing me. They wouldn't have raised that question if I had been experiencing a typical non-Christian Western allopathic healing, complete with white-coated doctors and drug prescriptions, because that's the way we Western Christians expect God to work. Jesus can do drugs but not Tai Chi. The newness of my circumstances waved red flags in their faces, and at that time I could not give them an answer. My halo was beginning to slip.

The questions increased when I purchased a book by a healer who sees the human energy field or "aura" in great detail and describes how she uses what she sees to heal others. I had taken a day-long course in therapeutic touch and wanted to do further investigation in energy healing. I ordered the book through a local seminary co-op at the same time I ordered a theology book. The store called and told me the theology book was in, and, since John, one of the members of our church and a very close friend, had his office in the same building on campus, I asked him to pick it up for me. "Sure, no problem." In the meantime, the "aura" book also came into the store without my knowledge. When John went to pick up the first book, the second was also there. He just handed me the bag and said absolutely nothing about the book, an indication of his discomfort with my purchase of it.

Not long afterward, John, who knew I had taken a course in therapeutic touch, sent me a conservative Christian magazine with a very deprecating article about it. The author described the practice as occurring in dimly-lit back rooms and as being ineffective, deceptive and spiritually dangerous because of its connection with "new age" ideas. It even mentioned that it might be "demonic." Of course, this did not match any of my experience or understanding of it. None of the healing I had experienced had occurred in dimly lit backrooms with deceptive practitioners but in my home and in Tai Chi classes with people who loved me and cared for me. I decided I needed to go to John and his wife Karen and have a talk with them.

Karen was one of my closest disciples, a woman whom I had mentored lovingly in prayer and ministry. She is the one who had brought it to the attention of the church that I was doing pastoral ministry even though I was seriously disabled. She and John both felt I was their spiritual mentor. Through my ministry they both experienced renewal and growth in their work. Besides that, we had shared years of joy and struggle in our personal lives. Our relationship had always been loving and warm. Now, as I entered their home, I sensed a cooler reception.

Hi Anna, come on in. Would you like some tea?"

"Sure," I said.

Karen went to the kitchen while John and I headed for the living room and chatted for a few minutes. Soon the tea appeared, and we began to sip the hot, herbal infusion as we transitioned to a more difficult topic.

"I wanted to get together with you and just see how you're feeling about things these days, about church and whatever is on your minds."

There was some hesitation in getting started, perhaps because we all knew there were things that they wanted to address but that would be uncomfortable for all of us. After all, I had been their mentor for some years, and it was hard for them to address questions about my actions and judgment.

Gradually they opened up.

"Well, Anna, "said John, "We don't understand about all the Tai Chi and therapeutic touch. I have some Chinese students, and when they come to Christ, Tai Chi and practices like that are some of the things they leave behind. We think it's okay to have healing that way, but it seems like you're kind of going a little too far with it. It seems like you're giving more honor to this fellow Bruce than you are to God." They were referring to my enthusiastic testimonies as my rehab progressed. I had shared my experiences openly, naively thinking everyone would be as happy as I was.

I encouraged them to continue talking so I could get a good idea of their feelings.

"This Eastern stuff you are doing, the meditation and all that, it isn't something we really feel comfortable with." They were referring to my introduction of some basic meditation practices into our cell group and church. I had been teaching people to sit quietly and meditatively, breathing and focusing on names of Christ. We had also done some visualization of bringing the Spirit in while inhaling and sending out disease and negative feelings while exhaling. All of it was done with Christian imagery. "That's just not the way we want to go," they said, "and we think it's dangerous for you. We're concerned about you. We don't want you to get involved in something that we think is too Eastern and not really centered on Christ."

It was almost as though I was standing outside the conversation, listening and observing. I could see their sincerity and their concern. Most of all I could see their deep love for me. They felt they were expressing something I needed to hear, and it was not easy for them to do so. I had always been the one to give them guidance, and now they wanted to help me. They were taking a stand for their own spiritual maturity, expressing their deeply held beliefs and concerns. They felt my soul was in jeopardy, and they were warning me as best they could. I recalled how all of my own children had done the same with their lives and decisions, and I felt the same conflicting emotions. There were feelings of hope and risk, pride and uncertainty, fulfillment and loss, all rolled into one. I wanted to hold on, and yet I also knew I needed to let go.

I wanted to pour my heart out to them, to tell them all my struggles—yes, the physical challenges, but especially the theological dilemmas I had been contemplating and working out with Shanta's help. I wanted to talk about the theological insights I was having and see how they could contribute to my understanding. But my experience and my theology were too new and raw. I couldn't even articulate them clearly to myself, much less someone else. I had no idea how to share in a way that would make sense in the daily life of our evangelical community.

I said, "God has done amazing things in my life, and I know it looks unusual from the outside. I don't know how to explain it. There are things I have experienced that I can't even talk about yet. I wish I could. I wish I could tell you everything."

"I don't see why you can't," John said.

I sat quietly for a moment, knowing I was in transition between two worlds, wondering if I could bridge the gap. Would they understand how I was trying to bridge the chasm between East and West at the same time I was working on rejuvenating a body that had been so engulfed by death? Would they have compassion for one so seriously disabled who found an amazing and yet strange path to healing? Would they feel I was fit to keep pastoring the church if I continued developing my new gifts and understanding? Would they find that my theological musings made sense, or would they reject them for more traditional interpretations that would squelch my new-born insights before I could fully examine them myself?

As we talked, I struggled back and forth with it and even opened my mouth to speak, but nothing came out. Finally, I knew in my heart it was too much. The reservations they were expressing were too deep, and I was not ready. It would take a long time of working together and studying together to come to a place where we could understand each other and where I would feel like I could share my experience fully. I decided I would ask them to join me on my journey. I said, "I don't understand everything that has happened, and it's going to take time for the understanding to come. I need to study and pray, and I need someone to help me with that. Will you help me explore the meaning of what has happened?"

Their heads were prayerfully bowed. After a time, John said, "Anna, that's not really the way we feel we want to go. What you're doing is just not in line with what we are trying to do with our ministry."

Karen was nodding her head, and tears were welling up in her eyes. She said, "Anna, in the past, you were the one who was always there for us and helping us when we needed it, but now you need us too. We're trying to let you know that we think this is not good for you."

I saw the depth of her feeling and sincerity. I said quietly, "I know you are sharing your hearts with me. Thank you for caring so much for me. But, you know, I don't feel I should stop what I'm doing now because it's bringing me such amazing healing. I believe with all my heart that what is happening to me is God's work and that Christ is at the center of it. And I believe that Tai Chi is God's way of helping me right now. Someday I will understand what it means and how to talk about it, but I don't right now."

"Anna, we love you, and we want you to know that we're not like those other people in your past who rejected you. We will pray for you and keep on loving you, but we just can't join you on this journey. We're on a different path."

Just as I had given my own biological children permission to go out in freedom and develop their own lives, I felt I needed to do that now with John and Karen. I didn't want them to feel that I was holding on to them or that I would make them feel guilty for their decision not to share my path. I wanted to set them free to develop their own ministry. I also wanted them to know that I believed God would take care of me. I would be okay.

I said, "I think this is an important day. I think you are saying to me that you want to follow God's guidance as you see best. I think what's happening here is that we're cutting the apron strings. I've been your mentor for a long time, and now you are ready to go on your own. That's a good thing! It's okay for us not to agree on this now. I know you love me and someday we'll all understand." Even as I said it, I felt a deep sorrow for what I knew could be the loss of their intimate friendship. We had shared so much in such precious love. I took a deep breath, took their hands into mine, and looked into their eyes. "I want you to know that I'm setting you free, with all my heart. I'm committing you to the way God has for you." The tears flowed as we prayed together that God would guide us all in the ways we would go.

I stepped out into the brisk night air, knowing things were changing, and I didn't know where it was all going. I felt disappointed that my friends were not able to walk with me through the healing that I knew was coming from God. I felt sad that they were not able to explore the meaning with me. Furthermore, I also knew that I was experiencing a change in status. I, who had been regarded almost as a "saint" while I was seriously disabled was now regarded as being on a "dangerous" path. My activities were considered strange and suspicious, even at the same time I was receiving the healing that my friends had prayed for so long. The healing just wasn't coming in the way any of us expected. I knew I would not give up my path of healing, and therefore I knew that my walk would be a lonely one. It would also be complicated by the fact that I was now in a pastoral position and would not be able to share either my progress or my questions with anyone in my congregation, except for Shanta. At the same time, the issues could not be hidden because my healing was progressing rapidly and visibly and could not be ignored.

In spite of all the questions, one thing was still very clear to me. Just as I had walked with Christ in that Picture on the Way years before, I was still walking with him. He was my center, my life, and nothing would ever change that. I could feel his strong presence, promising to guide me, and I knew he would, even when I didn't know where he was leading. I determined to go forward in faith, fixing my eyes on my Beloved.

I grew apart from John and Karen. I released them to pursue their ministry, and I pursued my own pastoring and the intense work of my healing. I shared less about my healing progress at church because I didn't want to offend people who didn't understand it. Gradually Karen became distant and aloof in my presence, barely able to speak to me. I didn't know what was going on, and I couldn't find out because John wasn't sharing with me either. In the coming months I would experience a lesson I had learned all too painfully in the past: deeply held religious beliefs are more powerful than the closest human bonds.

The Falling Icon

Not long after my conversation with John and Karen, I was exiting the door of a dorm on campus while Don was getting his coat on and chatting with some friends inside. We had just been attending the baby shower for our dear friends Dan and Anjie. As I stepped outside the door, I instinctively turned toward the handrail, which was two or three steps from the door to my right. Unfortunately, I didn't see that the top step on which I was standing was angled. My right foot went out into the air and found nothing there. Terrified, I knew I was in for a painful fall. I suddenly went into a dizzying space warp in which the normal physics of time and gravity were spinning crazily out of control. It seemed I was falling forever. In slow motion I felt my right leg buckling and my atrophied left leg trying to come forward but feeling slow, heavy and clumsy. My body was hurtling forward, my arms flying out, reaching desperately for the rail. The bags in my hand were floating slowly, noiselessly through the air. A cry from my throat seemed to fade in, grow to a crescendo, and then fade out again, like a train whistle passing in the night.

When I hit the concrete, I bounced and veered off backward and to the right. My right arm went up in protection but too late to keep my head from striking the side of the building. As the breath went out of me with a long whoosh, my body slid down the limestone façade and wedged tightly between the building and a decorative Ionic pillar. When I came to rest, my right arm and half of my body was hanging off the edge of the porch, and my other arm was pinned between my hips and the pillar. No one would ever believe that a person could land in such a distorted position. As I lay there dazed, it seemed like I entered a little space of eternity, a place where every thought, feeling, action and relationship was digitally framed, each byte of information capable of being paused, analyzed and edited. Even in the midst of pain, the events of the baby shower flashed through my mind.

What had gone amiss at the party? On the surface it was a joyous occasion, with our tightly-knit community coming together to celebrate the upcoming birth of a baby. Dan and Anjie were some of our closest friends. Both had attended the University of Chicago as undergrads and were now training to be doctors. They began to date while attending our cell group, and we shared each other's lives in the deepest sense. I had encouraged Anjie's poetical and musical expressions, and she had written numerous songs that were set to music by our worship team and were a part of the unique worship in our fellowship. Her deep prayer life gave her insights that undergirded her developing practice of ministry and medicine. She is the one who declared many months previously that I would have a Jubilee year, and she is the one who dreamed three times that I died and rose again. She told me once that my physical walk was a way of measuring what God was doing in my life. She recalled the Biblical story of the patriarch Enoch, who ascended and walked with God without experiencing death. She said, "One day, Anna, you will just rise up and walk and keep right on walking, all the way up." Anjie was a staunch ally and supporter for Don during his crises in the building of the Sloan Digital Sky Survey. Dan came from a family of ten children whose father was a well-known and beloved doctor in a nearby suburb. We shared with Dan the tragedy of his father's sudden death in an automobile accident on an icy freeway just before Christmas, and we were with him for the ensuing grief and reconstruction of his family. It seemed a friendship that was built on deep, solid foundations of mutual joy, suffering and sharing.

Other close friends were at the party as well. John and Karen seemed cordial on the surface but reserved underneath. They had not been the same since we had our talk. Marla was there with her husband Ted, and, as usual she had her guitar with her. Years before, I had encouraged her to write her own songs, and, as she experienced spiritual renewal, songs began to pour out of her, hallmarked by insight, originality and a deeply worshipful spirit. Marla was the powerhouse of creativity at the core of our church worship. Her husband Ted was a pianist and Bible teacher at the church for many years, and he was also musically creative.

Julia and Todd, who served as resident heads in the dorm, were putting on the shower, and we were using the dorm's party room. I had the feeling, after we were there for a short time, that the program of sharing and singing was already set. There was a little printed agenda of what would happen and some songs we would sing. Julia came to me and said, "Anna, would you like to read a scripture and say a prayer?"

"Of course," I replied. I noticed I was not on the agenda, but there was always a lot of flexibility in such things, and I didn't think anything about it at the time. I selected a passage that expressed my deep love for Dan and Anjie. Later, as I lay on the concrete and re-played the slo-mo video in my dizzied brain, it seemed like an afterthought when Julia asked me—more like the respectful but dutiful request of a pastor who happens to be on the scene than the loving and cherished inclusion of an old friend. When refreshments were served, I sat down on the floor in one of the circles, but I felt strangely out of the circle. My new duties and my intense rehab work were taking me out of the daily events of their lives. My new priorities and everyone's personal concerns and agendas were creating distance between us. These close friends were making reference to shared experiences that I didn't know about, and they had to explain to me what was going on. Conversation was courteous but lacked the comfortable warmth and humor that was so familiar from times past. It was confusing and unsettling. When it came my turn to read and pray, the response seemed once again to be dutiful, a marked change from previous times when my words would be warmly received as messages infused with Spirit.

Later, when the party was wrapping up, I picked up my dishes and said good-bye to those who were standing in small groups, still sharing the warmth of the occasion. There was a wave of some hands and "See you later," but no special hugs or prolonged conversation. I was free to go, but no one was accompanying me. That's when I headed for the door and stepped off the edge.

Now, as I lay on the concrete, no one knew I was in trouble. In that interminable moment, it seemed that the edge over which I had stepped was far more precipitous than I could have imagined. I was flying out into new territory, physically, spiritually, emotionally, relationally, and for all I knew I might land in some strange, impossible situation from which I could not extricate myself and from which no one could rescue me. My old familiar world seemed thin, tenuous and far away.

Soon Julia came out to say good-bye to someone, and she saw me wedged next to the building.

"Anna! Are you all right?!"

I couldn't answer. She loosened my arm and asked me if I could move, but I could not respond. She hurried inside to get Don.

Don rushed outside and knelt at my side.

"Anna, are you all right? Can you move? My eyes rolled and I groaned.

"Just lie still," he said, "until you feel okay. Shall I call an ambulance?"

The thought of making a scene like that seemed to hit me like cold water. "No, no! Just give me a moment."

As my eyes cleared, I said, "I think you can help me get out now."

It took two people to pull me free and then get me upright at the side of the pillar. Don supported me as I hobbled, bruised and bleeding, into the lobby and sat down heavily on one of the couches. Julia went into the party room a few paces away for some ice, which she brought to me in a plastic Ziploc bag. My friends knew I had fallen, but they were still inside chatting. In times past they would have gathered around me in loving support and prayer, but now it was just Don and Julia. Someone else came out of the room, and seemed to say from a thousand miles away, "Are you okay, Anna? I'm sorry you fell. I hope you're okay." Then she disappeared. I knew my friends well enough to know that even if it had been a stranger, they would normally have shown more concern than they were showing to me. Slowly, as I sat there recovering, the party broke up, and my friends filed past—John and Karen, Dan and Anjie, Marla and Ted. They waved their hands and said, "See you later. Hope you get to feeling better." No offers of help, no warm looks of support, no expressions of love and concern.

The contrast between the warmth of the past and the casual disregard of the present was like another wound, an invisible, internal wound, deep in my spirit. I had been held in high esteem, but now I was a falling icon. Don and I were the last to leave. As he helped me to the car, I was bruised and hurt. It was one of the loneliest trips I ever made.

Adventures and Vistas

It was the autumn of 2000, and Don and I were on our way home from China, an exotic adventure that even two years before I never would have dreamed I could take. Don was invited by Chinese astronomers to offer his expert advice about a new telescope they were planning to build and to pave the way for future joint scientific ventures with American astronomers. The Chinese gave us royal treatment. They paid all our expenses, including food and sightseeing, and provided a guide and chauffeured transportation everywhere we went. At the same time, they also shared their lives with us, and we saw that life in China during this time of explosive growth is not an easy one for the Chinese people. Even so, the trip was a happy, healing time for Don and me. It seemed that years of being enclosed in the small space of my home office were opening up to new possibilities as I reached out to try my new strength and energy in cities on the other side of the planet. We shared fun and adventure that had not been part of our lives for many years. We climbed the Great Wall, descended into the Ming tombs, and explored the Forbidden City and the Summer Palace on foot. We shopped in street bazaars and rode in bicycle taxis, and I even did Tai Chi at 6:00 a.m. in Heaven Temple. Don and I were both amazed at what I was able to do.

When Don was in meetings, Mr. Li, one of the most outgoing, joyous individuals I have ever met, would squire me around to any place I wanted to go, offering lively commentary and repartee along the way. Once he learned about my food needs and why I had such a strange diet, he took enthusiastic charge of all the ordering and made sure I had delicious vegetarian food for every meal. He took me shopping in street bazaars and

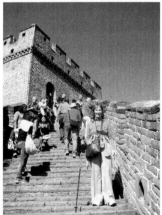

I can hardly believe it, but here I am at the Great Wall!

art stores. Once, when we were in a clothing store close to Tiananmen Square, he pulled a dress off the rack, all the while chatting rapidly in Chinese with the sales attendant. Then he spread the dress before me with a flourish and said, "She says you should try this one. You are very tall, and on you it will look very noble." Then his eyes twinkled and he said, "It's a sales tragedy." He was always trying new English words and was just getting them a little mixed up. Of course he meant sales "strategy." We laughed and laughed.

Mr. Li helped me purchase a very special piece of art that now hangs in my dining room. Everywhere I went in China I was looking for a traditional watercolor painting of plum blossoms, but I had not found one with just the right feeling about it. I was taking a rest in an art gallery one day, and as I sat there my eyes were roaming around the walls and alcoves. I caught sight of a plum blossom painting that for some reason stood out from any of the others I had seen. I liked the way the blossoms seemed to spring right out of the old, dead-looking branch. I said to Mr. Li, "Say, I really like that one there. Would you go ask that attendant about it?"

Mr. Li was soon in deep conversation with the sales lady. She was pointing out various features, and I saw Mr. Li expressing surprise and pleasure. Soon he came back grinning and looking like a cat that had swallowed a mouse. I wondered what he had discovered.

He said, "Oh Anna, it's a wonderful painting. The artist has painted it with special paint. During the cold, dry, winter season, only the darker blossoms show. But when the damper spring season comes, there is invisible paint that comes to life so that many more blossoms appear on the tree. And there is also a little bird that shows up on the end of the branch."

It was a kind of "living" piece of art! I knew that this painting was touching my heart. I looked at the inscription and wondered what the Chinese characters meant. I asked Mr. Li. He read it, and then waited a moment until he could translate it into appropriate English. With a glow in his voice, he said, "From the iron bone comes the spring."

I felt a gentle warmth flow through me. I knew that this painting was speaking to me of my own resurrection. My life had blossomed out of a branch that seemed as dead and cold as iron. Healing had come to me in the coldest, darkest time of my life, and now spring was coming. I purchased the treasure and carefully stowed it away to bring back home.

Along the way, as we saw the sites of Beijing, I shared with Mr. Li my journey from being a cripple to being able to make this trip. As he heard details of my story, he would get quiet and look at me in wonder. Once I saw tears in his eyes. His admiration grew as he saw how I plunged with such enthusiasm into each day's activities. Gradually I began to realize that everywhere we went he was telling people about me. Since he was speaking in Chinese, I didn't know what he was saying until those he was addressing would begin to look at me with wide eyes and nod their heads. Sometimes they would touch me softly, smiling and saying, "Ooh, ooh."

When it came time for us to leave for home, we felt we had never known such kind and hospitable people. As we parted at the airport, Mr. Li said, quietly and with deep sincerity, "You know, I am not a religious person, but almost you make me believe." My eyes filled with tears as I headed for the airplane, knowing my heart was connected with China and its people. In years to come, I would make more trips to China that would enrich my understanding of my own personal journey. I was beginning to experience deeply and personally the land that gave me gifts of healing.

The trip was not just a big step out into the world for me. It was also a time to bring closure to the most productive but painful period in Don's career. On the way home we were stopping in New Mexico for a couple of days to attend the dedication ceremony for the Sloan Digital Sky Survey. Don was the Founding Director for this cutting edge telescope, which was designed to map a large portion of the Universe. It was perched on the side of the mountain at Apache Point, a short distance away from the 3.5 meter telescope he had built in the

80's. A couple of smaller telescopes also peered out into space from there on the mountain, and the site was dotted with operations buildings and dormitories. Apache Point had become a center of observational astronomy that was changing the way we understand the Universe. Don had been like a father to it all, carefully tending it as it grew from a clearing in the forest to its current state. At this event he would see his dreams come to reality before his eyes, with astronomers and dignitaries from the many collaborating institutions there to celebrate their mutual achievement.

Even so, the event was bittersweet. Don was one of the visionaries who had conceived the project, and he had poured his life into it, fighting for funding, working through technological dilemmas, sorting out tangled personnel issues and refereeing fierce disagreements among his scientific peers. Don became so committed to the project that he felt the success of his whole career hung on it. He was devastated when he was removed from the directorship at a time when the project was in deep financial trouble. Even though he had already put in place the means of saving the project, he felt a terrible sense of failure and betrayal. From my side, I felt that Sloan was the project

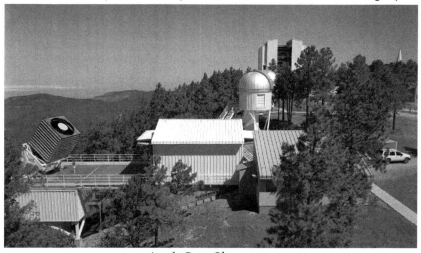

Apache Point Observatory:
Don was the Founding Director of The Sloan Digital Sky Survey (left)
and the 3.5 meter telescope (rear right).

that nearly destroyed our marriage. The dedication ceremony was an event that we hoped would help bring closure to a long and difficult time in our lives.

We arrived after the ceremony began. Part of the reason was that I had an acute case of *tourista* and we had to stop the car every few miles so I could run to the restroom. Another reason was that traveling up the mountain with the brilliant colors of autumn splashing the hillsides was a sentimental journey, bringing back memories of the time we had lived there and the adventures we had shared. We didn't hurry on our drive. When we passed the ranch at midpoint, I remembered clearly the night I had been trapped on the mountain during a snowstorm. With each turn of the road and with each new vista, old memories came flooding back. As we approached Apache Point, I had mixed emotions. This would be the first time I had seen the telescope that had consumed so much of Don's life. We parked our rental car and waited for a shuttle to take us from the main road to the telescope area. That took more time than we expected. When we arrived, I realized we were not just a few minutes late. Somehow Don had not accurately remembered the starting time, and the speeches were already well underway. I looked at him with question marks. He shrugged his shoulders and rolled his eyes.

We collected our sweatshirts and folders and took a seat in the back of the crowd. The sky was a brilliant blue, as it can only be in the Land of Enchantment, and the air was crisp and full of the scent of pine. Representatives of the various collaborating institutions, including Princeton University, Johns Hopkins, the University of Chicago, and the University of Washington gave speeches, noting the remarkable achievement and the scientific breakthroughs that were expected to come from the new telescope. Later, we learned we missed the speech in which Don was especially honored. We watched as the dignitaries lined up to cut the ribbon and cheered along with everyone else as the telescope was officially launched on what would become a brilliant, paradigm-breaking career.

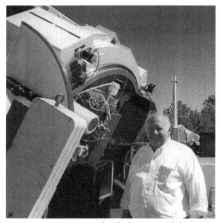
2000: Don at the dedication of the Sloan Digital Sky Survey.

When the ceremony ended, it seemed that the ice broke for Don. He took his position at the telescope, joyously describing its features to many friends and colleagues and basking in the success of the event. Many people noted with admiration his role in the project.

That evening at the banquet in The Lodge, the historic mountain retreat in Cloudcroft, we heard the words we needed to hear, words that would heal us and help us move on with our lives. After citing the contributions of many different people and institutions, the current Director of the project said, "And now I want to say that there are many people who have contributed to this project. But without one certain individual and his years of commitment and sacrifice, this telescope would never have come into being. He was there from the beginning and he saw the project through some of its most difficult days. He is the Founding Director of the Sky Survey." He turned to look at Don. "Don York, without you we wouldn't be here celebrating tonight. From all of us here, we thank you from the bottom of our hearts."

Don stood, and there was a long round of loud, warm applause that surrounded us like healing balm. The future seemed to be opening new vistas to us and saying, "Yes, now you can begin to live again."

Rising Costs

As it turned out, we were not able to bask too long in the glow of fulfillment. Our good feelings and our hearts were shattered the next morning when I made a call home and Shanta broke some bad news about our church.

"Hey Shanta," I said as he answered on the Chicago end.

"Oh, Anna! Are you back?"

"Well, we soon will be. We just finished the dedication ceremony at Apache Point. We'll be home tonight. How are things going?" I was eager to catch up on the latest news.

"Well," he said, "a lot of things have changed since you left. I didn't want to ruin your trip, so I decided to wait till you came back."

I caught my breath, fearing a death or serious illness. "So what's going on?"

"Well, the Sunday after you left, a whole lot of people just didn't show up for church. They all decided they aren't coming back."

I waited in silence a moment, then asked, "Who was it?" even though I thought I knew.

"Several of the core people," he said with a strained voice. He named all of those who had been my closest friends, Ted and Marla, John and Karen, Dan and Angie and their families. He wasn't sure, but he thought some others could possibly be leaving soon as well.

I felt a hard knot form in my midsection. "I see. So did they say why they were leaving?"

"Anna, I'm not really surprised. I think we've known that they are angry about the way we've handled things recently. I think they just decided they would make as strong a statement as they could by leaving."

I was overwhelmed by sadness. We talked a little longer, and then Don and I had to leave to catch our plane in Albuquerque. We agreed we would talk when we arrived in Chicago.

As we drove that four-hour trip through the desert, my heart seemed to match the landscape—dry and stony. I rehashed the last several months in my mind, trying to put the pieces together into a picture that made sense. Yes, there had been a crisis that had rumbled like an earthquake through our church. The pastoral team spent untold hours working with those involved, but some core members who had been my close friends strongly disagreed with the pastoral decisions. Fingers pointed, gossip circulated, and the church began to break into factions.

That crisis was not the only issue we faced. Some of same people who were involved in the emotional turmoil were dissatisfied with their roles in the church. Once I became stronger physically, there was less reticence about critiquing my performance. I was somehow more "human," and less saintly now that I seemed to be experiencing success and gaining physical strength. Some thought I was a better minister when I was disabled and even seemed to be wistful about "the good old days." It almost seemed that my previously serious illness had been a catalyst by which people could sublimate their personal traumas, holding them in abeyance in respect for one whose problems were obviously so much greater than their own. I was an opportunity for heroic Christian endeavor—until my own heroic endeavors began to shine so brightly in healing and strength and a new life. Unexpected anger began to break out toward me, anger I did not understand and could not address.

My relationship with John and Karen deteriorated. When Karen came to church and prayer meetings, she was unable to look at me or speak to me. Finally, I stopped her one Sunday after church and said, "Please, Karen, talk to me. What's going on? How can we resolve this situation?"

With great difficulty and without looking me in the eye, she said, "Anna, you've been angry with me for months." I was shocked because I was not aware of feeling anger toward her. I knew there was a serious miscommunication, and I wanted to heal it with this person who was so dear to me. "Can we get together and talk about that? I'd liked to clear it up. Could we meet together?" She was deeply hurt and could hardly bear to stand and talk with me, but she agreed to meet.

In the meantime, I searched my heart for any feelings of anger I might have against her. I also asked Don and Shanta if they had any impression from our conversations that I was angry toward Karen. No, they didn't have any idea that was the case. I thought perhaps she was taking some of the things I said in my sermons personally, but I wasn't sure what it would be. While pondering these things, I suddenly remembered the big clash she had with Sifu Bruce at the wedding of my oldest son. Bruce had been moving the gift table inside the reception hall to protect the gifts from potential theft, when Karen confronted him angrily and insisted that the table remain where it was. She was in charge, and she wanted it done her way. Fireworks went off, and the air was still charged when I arrived on the scene a short time later to resolve the dispute. I saw that she was angry with Bruce beyond the small matter that triggered the explosion. I suspected that she regarded him as the person who was taking me away, not only from her and my other friends, but also, in her view, enticing me away from God. She was worried about my soul, and she saw him as the enemy she needed to confront. She did it there over the gift table.

Karen and I had two meetings, and they did not go well. I tried to fill in the gaps so she would know what my life had been like and that I was not angry with her. I said, "You know, after the meeting I had with you and John, I was sad, but I understood your feelings. You said you would pray for me, and I knew you would. I had to move on with my life. I was very busy working with my new responsibilities at church, and I was also doing intense rehab on my body. My mother died, and that consumed a lot of my time and emotional energy, and then there was the wedding. And all this time, I've been trying to come to terms with what has happened to me. You know, Karen, I wasn't angry with you. I just had so much going on in my life."

"Anna," she said, "for me you were such a spiritual guide. I held you in such high esteem. You taught John and me so much. You changed our lives and showed us how to do such beautiful ministry. And now…." Here her voice wavered and her eyes looked down. "We love you, and, well, you abandoned us." Then her voice was shaking with emotion. "Anna," she said, "You need us. You need us in your life. We want to be there for you. We don't know what you're doing. We don't know what to do."

I recalled the terrible fall I had taken the day of the baby shower and how everyone seemed to pass by without helping me. I stopped her for a moment and asked her, "What happened that day of the shower, Karen, the day I fell and everyone seemed to ignore me."

She knew what I was talking about. She said, "You know, Anna, none of us knew if you would want our help. So we didn't do anything." Frozen in uncertainty and frustration, their behavior had come across as uncaring and hurtful.

She went on. "We felt like you were such a saint, and we hung on your every word. We would do anything for you. But now, you've betrayed us!" Tears streamed down her face. "Now we see that Saint Anna can not only be wrong—she can be *very* wrong!" Her hurt came pouring out. I saw that in her eyes I was indeed an idol that had fallen from its ivory pedestal. I was no longer a saint but a human being with flaws and struggles like everyone else. She was mourning the loss of a beautiful and profound relationship that was built on a myth I could not sustain. There was also the confusing experience of praying for so long and fervently for my healing, of envisioning it and believing in it—and then having it turn out so differently from what was expected. There was no healing at the altar! How did Tai Chi get in there! All of that Eastern stuff was unfamiliar and even scary. It wasn't supposed to happen that way!

But it seemed that perhaps the cruelest cut of all was that I had new friends and no longer seemed to need my old friends as I once did. I was spending time with other people and was not heeding the sincere words of warning that they felt were coming from God. The words "you abandoned us" and "you betrayed us" were spears in my heart. I knew that along with feelings of abandonment and betrayal come anger and distrust. If we were to overcome this barrier between us, it would take a long time and a lot of hard work. I declared my willingness to do the work, but I saw it would be delayed for months by their summer travel and our trip to China. Even with the deepest commitment, it would be a long, painful healing.

I thought of all these things as we drove through the desert, mile after mile, heading for Albuquerque. The weather was unsettled. We watched as the clouds formed shifting dark patches on the desert floor. We could see the storm clouds forming at a distance, watch them approach closer and closer, flashing lightning, and then feel the car shake as we were engulfed by wind-driven rain.

It was a long trip home, and when we arrived we found a church in shock and grief. Our friends did not say good-bye to the church or request the traditional prayers we always offered to those who were leaving our fellowship. They just left and never came back. Gossip flew around, a secret letter was passed, and fingers pointed in all directions. More families left, some in sympathy with their friends, some because the situation was difficult, and some because they felt I was setting a bad example by doing Tai Chi. Some hoped to make a strong statement of dissatisfaction and, perhaps, to provoke us to repentance for things they considered "wrong." There were angry, prophetic statements of doom.

The reasons for the crisis were many and complex, and I have not been able to sort through it to find any answer other than the prayerful path we took. Even so, I still cannot help but feel that my friends might have stuck it out longer and tried to work things out if only I had been able to find some way to help them understand what I was going through.

In the ensuing months, we struggled to bring healing to our fractured community. I was thankful for those faithful, hearty souls who endured the transition in which we re-visioned who we were as a church. We changed our affiliation from Southern Baptist to the more liberal and inclusive Alliance of Baptists, created a new name and identity for our church, and set ourselves on a new path of mission and ministry.

I struggled with my own personal brokenness. I talked with Shanta, attended communication training sessions and read various books, exploring how I had failed and how I could grow in the future so such things did not happen again. I learned a lot, but I did not come up with any easy answers. I learned that when I am experiencing such profound transformation, it is necessary to bring loved ones along as gently but as openly as possible. Some of them will hang in there, weather the changes, and be part of a new life. Some will continue to love me, even though they think I am on the path to perdition. And some, no matter how much I might try, will leave my life forever.

I discovered that rifts in relationships are characteristic of people who experience massive changes in their lives, including near-death and healing experiences such as my own. During the course of survival and recovery, choices must be made and priorities must change. Some of the people who are the most loving and who take the most personal responsibility for another person's health and wellbeing find it difficult to step back and allow that person to make decisions that seem risky or even dangerous. That happened with my doctor who warned me about stopping the drugs; it happened with Don when he begged me to keep using my cane; it happened with my friends and some family members who were concerned about my immortal soul. It almost seems that the more people care and the longer they are involved the more strongly they state their concerns so that their behavior may come across as angry, demanding and frustrated. The more deeply they care, the more they are hurt when their life giving advice is not heeded. The more crucial role they have played, the more devastated they are when they sense they are no longer needed in the same way. Transformation has a high price tag. Relationships cannot be freeze-framed and hung on the wall to admire. They are dynamic and changing. Even the strongest relationships can suffer irreparably.

As Don and I talked about it, he said to me, "Anna, you have to understand that you're not like most people. Other people pretty much keep going on with the same kind of life they've always lived.

You keep on changing. When you get knocked down, you get up and keep on going. That's kind of threatening for a lot of people, including me. We don't know what to do with it. We just want to keep living our normal lives."

I let out a deep breath and went into his arms for a tender hug. "I don't know about other people, Honey, but I guess that's the way I am." I rested my cheek against his broad chest and recalled how he has always been there for me. He was there at the birth of all five of our children, and he helped bury one of them. He was there as a loving, hands-on father, changing diapers, taxiing kids to sports activities, paying the bills for college. He was there through all the years of my illness, doing the jobs of two parents, keeping his career going and holding the family together. And during the years of my healing, even when all my changes were disrupting his life and he didn't understand what I was doing, he was still there. What an awesome man! A lesser man would have been gone long ago. Tears came to my eyes and thanksgiving washed over me for my heart's companion, the most amazing gift God has given me in my life.

After a few moments, I said, "Well, there's one thing I know."

"Yeah?"

"I know you love me. You've been with me all the way. Even through all the changes and all the hardest times, for almost 40 years, you've always been there."

"Mmhmm. And I always will be," he said huskily.

I remembered the song we had sung to each other almost every year on our anniversary: "I love you more today, more today than yesterday, and I love you less today, less than I will tomorrow." We cherished the moment.

Finally, I said, "It's been a long time, and I still have a lot to do. I still have to learn how to walk so I don't fall on my face."

"In more ways than one!" he said.

"Ha ha," I responded. Then I continued, "And I still don't know what it all means. I need to be able to tell my story. It seems like the day I stop growing will be the day I'm ready to leave this place. It's grow or die, baby. Can you handle that?"

He rolled his eyes in mock horror. Then he tightened his arms around me and grinned. "We've come this far. It would be a shame to quit now."

Photo Album

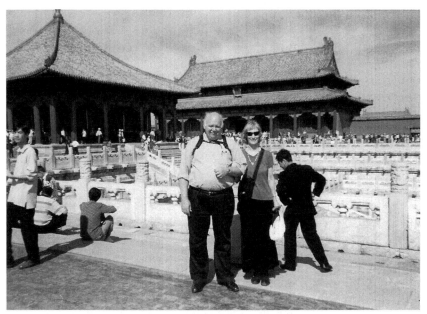

Forbidden City in Beijing, China, 2000.

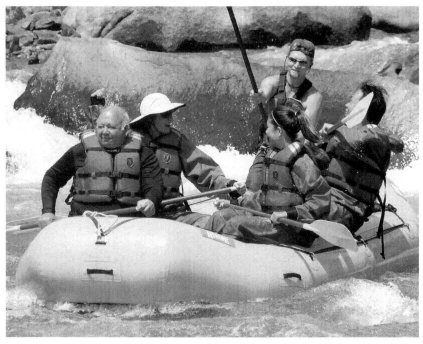

Whitewater rafting in Colorado, 2004.

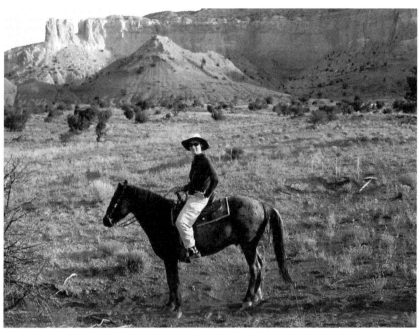

Anna at Ghost Ranch, New Mexico, 2007

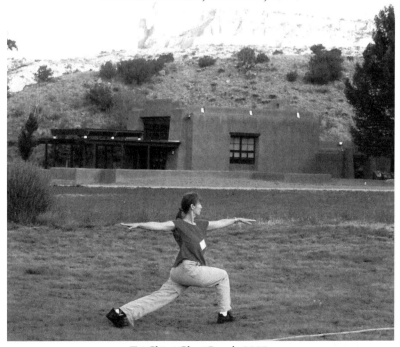

Tai Chi at Ghost Ranch, 2007.

Photo Album

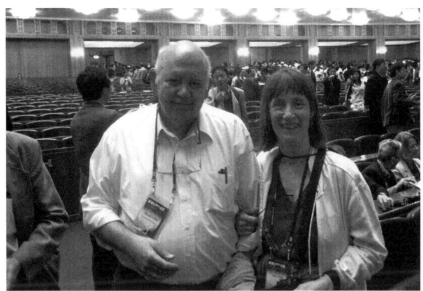

Don and Anna at the Great Hall of the People in Beijing after opening ceremonies for the NV400 Conference celebrating the invention of the telescope. Don was the organizer of the conference. Four Nobel Laureates spoke at this event, which was attended by 7000 top high school students from Beijing.

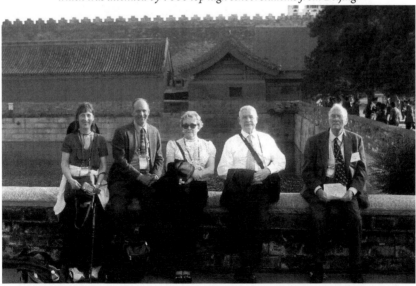

Outside the Forbidden City, 2008, with speakers at the NV400 Conference: Anna, Geoffrey Marcy, Winner of the Shaw Prize for discovery of planets around stars; Mrs. Ricardo Giacconi; Ricardo Giacconi, Nobel Laureate in Physics; Charles Towns, Nobel Laureate in Physics and inventor of the laser.
We crossed the Forbidden City in 30 minutes with Charlie, at age 94, leading the way.

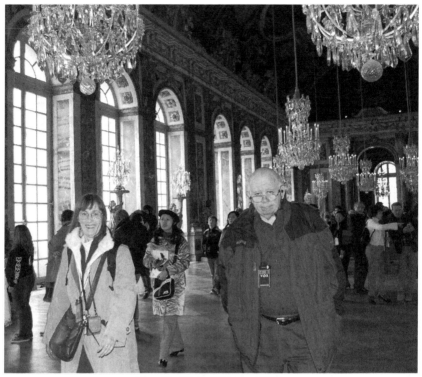
Versailles Hall of Mirrors, 2008.

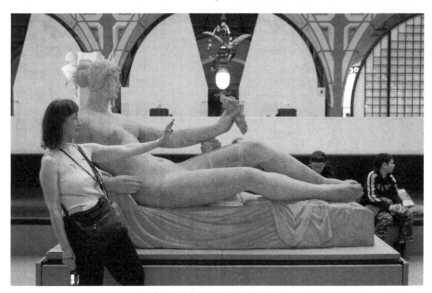
Orsay Museum, Paris, 2008.

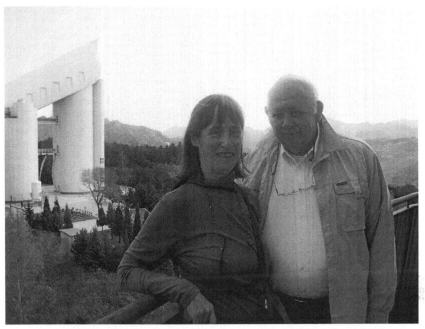

Don and Anna at the Dedication of the Xinglong Obsevatory in China, 2008.

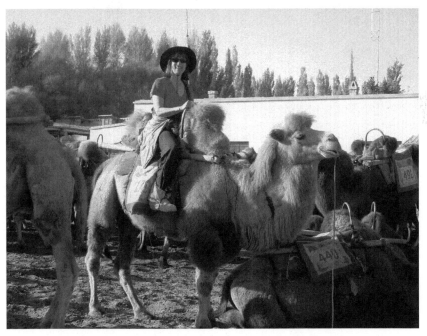

Camel riding at the Singing Sands in the Gobi Desert, 2008.

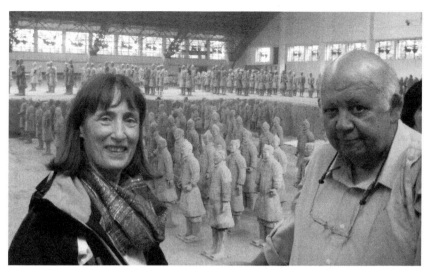

Visiting the Terracotta Soldiers at Xian, China, 2008.

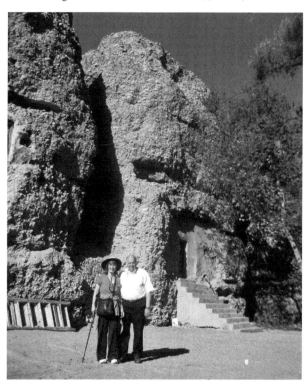

Don and Anna at the 10,000 Buddhas Caves in the Gobi Desert, 2008. The caves are near the site of the discovery of ancient texts describing the early Chinese Church.

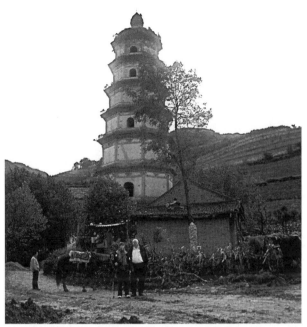

Don and Anna at Da Qin Pagoda, the remains of the first Chinese Church, established in 635 a.d.

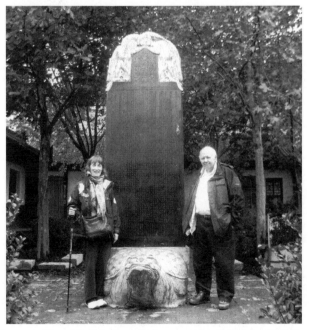

The stone stele at Da Qin that tells the story of early Chinese Christians.

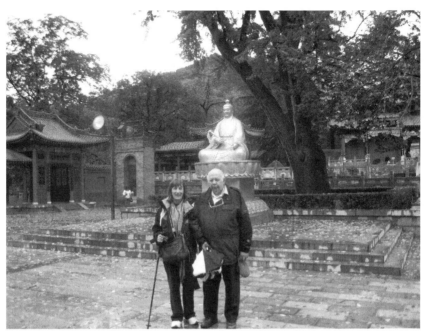

Lou Guan Tai, the ancient monastery where Lao Tzu wrote the Tao te Ching, is on a mountain across the valley from Da Qin.

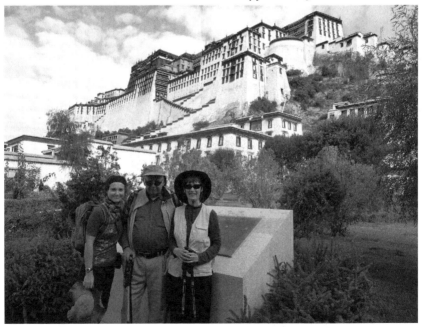

Emily, Don and Anna York at the Potala Palace in Lhasa, Tibet, 2009.

Photo Album

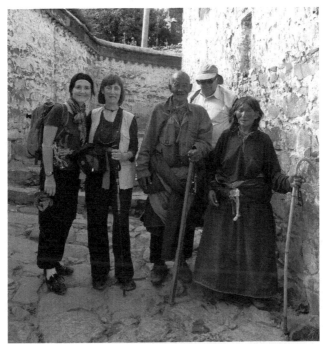

With Tibetan nomads at a mountain monastery in Tibet, 2009.

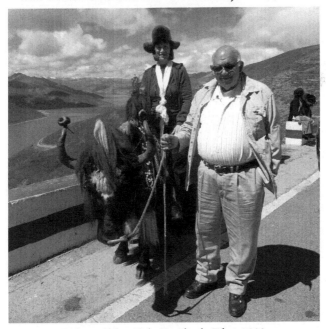

Riding a Yak at Lake Yamdrock, Tibet, 2009.

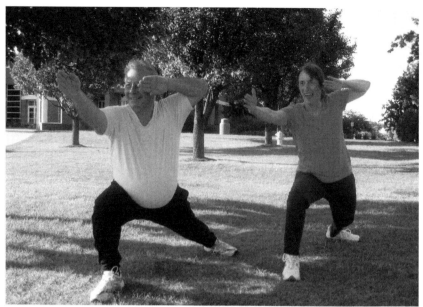
Tai Chi with Sifu Ed Gierut, 2009.

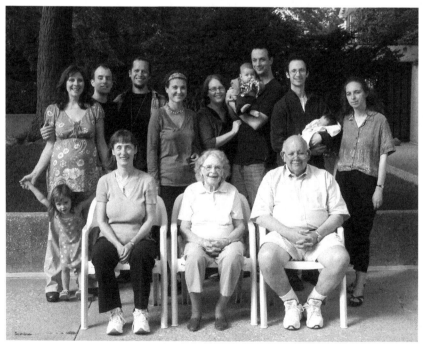
York family reunion in 2008. Our clan is growing!

Epilogue

Epilogue

New Year, 2010

Today is the first Sunday of a new year and a new decade. It is almost ten years since the trip to China and the fracturing of our church community that created such heartbreak, ten years of rehabbing my body and my life, ten years of changing and healing relationships, ten years of growing, becoming.

It is so appropriate that Don and I should spend this day with Shanta, who has had such a great impact on my life and my healing. Shanta and his wife Dhilanthi are back in town for their daughter's wedding. We have now been friends for over twenty years, evidence that through all of our trials some relationships not only endure but flourish with time.

This morning we are all going back to that same church where we marked out significant mileposts on our life journeys. Shanta is invited to speak and tell about his work as the Director of Inter-Religious Dialogue and Cooperation for the World Council of Churches. Shanta is the man who has the leading global voice for Protestant Christian churches in relation to other religions in the world. He is an ardent activist for cooperation, justice and peace where there is often bloody conflict. I could have asked for no better mentor as I sorted out the meaning of a healing that came from a radically different culture and philosophy than my own conservative Christian background.

After Shanta left his pastorship in Chicago, I also found it necessary to move on so new leadership could come into the church. We have kept good friendships there, but I have not visited a worship service for some years. I am looking forward to hearing what Shanta has to say and to seeing how the church is faring.

We are greeted at the door with a bustle of energy from a large number of African Ameri-

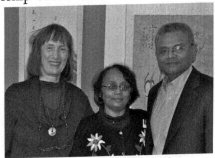

New Year, 2010: Anna with Dhilanthi and Shanta.

can teens, talking animatedly in pairs and small groups, waiting for the service. The sanctuary fills up fast, partly with guests to hear Shanta, but also with current members of the church. It is obvious in an instant that this church continues to be the most diverse church I have ever experienced, represented by all races and socio-economic groups. I take my seat and look around. The vibrant spirit lets me know that God is alive and well in this church, a fact that receives strong emphasis when a gospel choir of fourteen youth exuberantly sings "Down by the Riverside."

As the youth sing, my fingers touch the blue fabric of the chairs, and I remember when I selected the chairs and ordered them in the early 90's. The music continues, and it seems that a cloud gently begins to fill the space, a shimmering, palpable delitescence in which temporal dimensions mingle together so that past, present and future are all present in one luminous, infinite moment. All I have ever experienced in that place is there with me as I begin to recall stories and people behind the pictures on the wall, the banner hanging in the window, the podium tapestry, the carpeting on the floor, even the paint on the walls. Beyond the physical, there is, so to speak, a "cloud of witnesses"—all the people we have known, the times we have shared, the friends who have come and gone, the life events of marriage, death and healing, the joys, the hurts, the struggles, the triumphs. I see my soul as integrally infused with this place.

Present in heart and spirit are my immediate family members, the four sons who grew up in this church, now all grown and married to very special women who have helped balance out the historical male predominance in the family. For so many years I held my own with five men in the house! I have had the joy of performing the marriage ceremonies for three of my sons—Sean to Emily, Maurice to Dasa, and Chandler to Kara. Shanta officiated for Jeremy and Elisa's wedding while I enjoyed the first of my sons' weddings as Mom. Jeremy's wedding reception was held here in this room. We are now the proud grandparents of four grandchildren, and I am living a life with them that I dared not dream of fifteen years ago. In the dark days when I could not even think of tomorrow, I certainly could not envision enjoying my grandchildren. Now I can play with them, read to them and participate actively in their lives—and I hope to do so for many years to come. My cup overflows.

As Shanta begins to speak, it seems that the Spirit opens spaces between the words, windows into my soul. It was here in this church where so many prayers ascended for me from hearts and hands of love. Yes, there was a breach in those loving relationships, a rift I thought might never be healed. Certainly I had no plan or vision for how it could happen after all of my friends left the city and moved to far distant places. But time and grace do their work. In 2008, eight years after the explosion in our community, a miracle happened in my heart. I was able to reach out to all of them, asking forgiveness and seeking a renewal of relationships. They all responded, and now the shadows of hurt have lifted from my heart—and I hope from theirs. We can never go back and make it like it was before, but we can move forward, and that is a miracle. I am so grateful that my love and prayers can go out joyously to them.

It was in this room, at that very same podium, that I was ordained to ministry, and some of those who were present then are here today, twelve years later. Peggy, Brenda, Hill and Cheryl all laid hands of blessing on me, and Shanta preached that memorable sermon about pouring tea. Dhilanthi's arrangement of my songs infused them with a vibrancy far beyond my humble words and music.

Bruce Moran, my teacher for fourteen years, still does his healing, therapy and training practice in downtown Chicago. I am deeply grateful that he was there for me for so many years, helping me return to health and vitality. Other Tai Chi friends who were present at my ordination have all moved on, and I am always delighted to hear from them as they experience various life events. They played a powerful, crucial role in my life, and I am forever changed by their friendship, their wisdom and their skill. Whenever I do Tai Chi or Chi Kung, I still hear their voices, correcting, encouraging and inspiring. They are a blessing.

Don of course is present today as he always has been. Don is still living up to his motto, "Make no small plans." The Sloan Digital Sky Survey that caused us so much pain in the 1990's has now become the most successful astronomical mapping project ever launched and has been dubbed by *Scientific American* as one of the seven wonders of modern astronomy. The thousands of scientific papers that have been generated from SDSS data by scientists around the world provide some satisfaction for the years of turmoil that were required to bring it to birth and launch it into service. Don continues to write prolifically and travels often to China to work on international projects. I sometimes accompany him. He is still the Executive Director of CUIP, the computer installation-and-training program that serves about 30 schools in neighborhoods surrounding Hyde Park.

As for me, I cannot help comparing the person I was at my ordination to the person I have become. I look at the podium and recall that I was barely able to stand there for my ordination address. Now I am strong and I live an active, vibrant life. Even though my chronological age is relentlessly rising, my functional age still seems to get younger as I enjoy more energy and stamina. I still have weakness in my lower left side, but it doesn't keep me from working, teaching classes, walking, hiking in the mountains with my trekking poles and doing Tai Chi to my heart's content. Recent physical exams testify that I am healthy all around. After a quarter century of being uninsurable, I am now healthy enough to qualify for life insurance! Don jokes that I am now worth something when I die.

It was here in this church that I pondered the dilemma of my Chinese/Tai Chi healing as it relates to Christianity. I have vigorously pursued answers and will continue to do so. Don and I have even traveled to the far corners of China to discover the roots of the ancient Chinese Church that was established there in 635 A.D. and was then lost to history a few hundred years later. These theological explorations and travel adventures are a great story in themselves, one that I hope to share in due time.

The Tai Chi and Chi Kung that were so strange to me before have become highly relevant to my Christian spiritual life and practice. A few years ago, Sifu Bruce authorized me to teach Chi Kung, which I have developed into a form that I call New Creation Body Prayer. It employs the nature imagery and movements of traditional Chinese Tai Chi Tao and Chi Kung forms that have stood the test of time and that are being practiced by millions of people around the world today for their health benefits. I have put them together with Judeo-Christian imagery in a Genesis Creation Story setting that makes the Chinese practice accessible and spiritually relevant for Westerners—and especially for Christians. I also teach a secular form of the same movements. I teach classes in a rehabilitation hospital and in a rehab sports facility in downtown Chicago, as well as classes in the Hyde Park and Beverly neighborhoods. I feel deeply gratified that I am able to share the wonderful healing movements with those who have a great variety of disabilities, including multiple sclerosis. My heart is full of thanksgiving as I see many of my students experience some of the healing benefits that have been so important for me.

I understand now that Christ has guided me on a journey of bridge building that was not just for my own benefit. I have built a healing bridge between East and West that I could not previously have traveled myself. Hope is the most precious commodity to those who are in pain and despair. Where there is no hope, the past is bitter, the present unbearable, the future unthinkable. I have built a bridge of hope. I hope many will cross over and find healing and wholeness.

Shanta's voice calls me back from my reverie, and I realize the service has moved on. As the congregation sings and claps the final song, the vitality of the voices and the heartbeats of those around me cause that ever-present "cloud of witnesses" to evanesce before my spiritual eyes. As the benediction is spoken, I capture a brief, shimmering vision of all those who have gone before, spreading their hands of blessing and guiding us into the future.